ISBN: 9781696889360

An original work published in 2019 by:

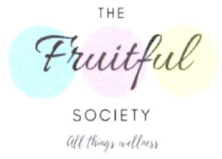

▶ YouTube

Go to You Tube and search for "The Fruitful Society" to view the following 3 video commentaries which will enhance your understanding of this research report.

- Basics to "A radical theory on men metabolic syndrome/ infertility (MetS) & Depression"

- Impaired men metabolic syndrome/ infertility (MetS) symptoms and reasons

- Depression in men (BPD/Dysthymia/Bipolar/Major) symptoms and reasons

Legal disclaimer: This report (including any associated contents) is not intended to replace the services of a doctor, nor does it constitute a doctor-patient relationship. Information is provided for informational purposes only and is not a substitute for professional medical advice. You should not use the information here to diagnose or treat a medical or health condition. If you have or suspect you have an urgent medical problem, promptly contact your professional healthcare provider. Any application of the recommendations from this report or its associated contents is at the reader's discretion.

A radical theory on men metabolic syndrome/infertility (MetS) & Depression (BPD/Borderline, Dysthymia, Bipolar, Major)

Section	Description	Page No.
	Introduction	1
A	Stress and its relationship with energy levels:	3
	i. Energy intake	3
	ii. Energy redirection & amplification of mental resilience and intimidating physical features	3
	• Aromatization	5
	iii. Over exertion of energy countered by nutritional & mental coping methods	8
	iv. Men metabolic syndrome/ infertility (MetS) case study	16
	v. Men metabolic syndrome/ infertility (MetS) symptoms & root causes	17
	vi. BPD or Borderline depression case study	19
	vii. BPD or Borderline depression symptoms & root causes	20
	viii. Dysthymia case study	23
	ix. Dysthymia symptoms & root causes	24
	x. Bipolar case study	25
	xi. Bipolar symptoms & root causes	26
	xii. Major depression with anxiety case study	27
	xiii. Major depression with anxiety symptoms & root causes	28
	xiv. Men metabolic syndrome/ infertility (MetS) with BPD or Borderline depression case study	29
	xv. Men metabolic syndrome/ infertility (MetS) with Dysthymia case study	31
	xvi. Men metabolic syndrome/ infertility (MetS) with Bipolar case study	33
	xvii. Men metabolic syndrome/ infertility (MetS) with Major depression with anxiety case study	35
	xviii. Common root causes and impaired body mechanism between 'Men metabolic syndrome/ infertility' and Depression	36
B	Stress & free radical damages:	37
	• Impact leading to impairment/diseases (i.e. Men metabolic syndrome/ infertility (MetS), Depression (i.e. Borderline Personality Disorder (BPD) or Borderline, Dysthymia, Bipolar, Major)	
C	Problems in neutralizing free radical damages:	39
	i. Impaired methylation and its impact	39
	ii. Depleted glutamine level and its impact	41
D	Impact of stress on the neuroendocrine functions:	45
	i. Metabolic issues (insulin resistance, increasing triglycerides, protein depletion from muscles, diabetes, thyroid problems, central obesity, acne)	45
	• Hydroxylation	47
	ii. Hormonal imbalance (low sex drive, fertility issues, sexual dysfunction, sperm production problems, feminization)	48
	iii. Weak cholesterol profile (cholesterol plagues, cardiovascular problems, high blood pressure, kidney problems)	50
	iv. Lowered bile movement or bile sluggishness (bad bacteria build up, gut issues, toxin build up, liver fat, vision problems, weak immunity, infertility, inflammation, skin health issues, bruising)	52
	v. Impaired detoxification (toxin build up, imbalance hormone & neurotransmitter level)	52
E	Impact of nutrition to prevent or heal from a neuroendocrine imbalance	54

Section	Description	Page No.
F	Depression & Neurotransmitters	57
	i. Neurotransmitters	57
	i-1: Emotional mental stress, neurotransmitter over signalling, free radical attacks to brain, depression	58
	• Hydroxylation and oxygen deprivation in the brain	58
	• Major depression with anxiety chart	59
	i-2: Chronic emotional mental stress, brain neurotoxin, resistant depression	60
	• BPD/Borderline depression (splitting) chart	61
	• Bipolar charts	62
	• Dysthymia chart	63
	i-3: Effective methylation, hydroxylation and oxygen level in the brain to prevent depression	63
	• A rebalanced brain chart	63
	ii. Neurotransmitters (brain chemicals) spectrum of emotions & functions	64
	• GABA (Degree of Calmness)	64
	• Oxytocin (Degree of Focus)	64
	• Glutamate (Degree of Alertness)	66
	• Serotonin (Degree of Wellbeing)	66
	• Dopamine (Degree of Drivenness)	67
	iii. Why Depression & Mania happens	68
G	Case study: Major depression with anxiety, BPD/Borderline depression, Bipolar and Dysthymia	72
H	Summary of depression neurotransmitter profiles	76
I	Neurotransmitter imbalance and ways to rebalance	77
J	Inconsistent findings on testosterone therapy in relieving depression	80
K	Common concise protocol & nutrient intake to rectify 'Men metabolic syndrome/ infertility' (MetS) and Depression (BPD/Borderline depression, Dysthymia, Bipolar and Major depression with anxiety)	82
L	Implications for physical and mental health	85
	Acknowledgement	86
	Appendix 1: Links	87

Introduction

The prevalence of metabolic syndrome (MetS) is increasing worldwide almost approaching the pandemic state. Its key components, namely, obesity, insulin resistance, dyslipidemia, and hypertension can have detrimental effects on various aspects of human health. Male fertility is one condition that can be influenced by MetS through several mechanisms. Endocrine system dysregulation, scrotal temperature elevation, oxidative stress, and alteration of the erectile and ejaculatory functions are well recognized MetS consequences that can impair sperm production and function, ultimately affecting male fertility. A healthy lifestyle characterized by good nutrition and regular physical activity is key to prevent the unwanted effects of MetS not only on fecundity but also on health and well-being overall, excerpt from article (Link 1) and (Link 2).

According to the articles here, (Link 3), (Link 4), (Link 5) and (Link 6), there is a relationship between depression and metabolic syndrome.

Both MetS and depression are complex diseases and the world has yet to discover the real reasons they arise.

Problems with the current global research: There is a research silo between conventional/ naturopathic/ neuroscience/ psychology/ endocrine and mental health fields. Metabolic syndrome (MetS) and Depression (i.e. Borderline Personality Disorder (BPD)/Borderline, Dysthymia, Bipolar and Major depression) are body-wide problems. Currently, the research merely lists the constellation of symptoms within each disorder, however, the symptoms interrelationships within each disorder respectively and the interrelationships between MetS and the depressive disorders are unknown.

Objectives of this report: To discover the real reasons behind MetS, BPD/Borderline, Dysthymia, Bipolar and Major depression along with their interrelationships, to better quantify /measure the disorder in order to find actionable natural solutions to healing. There should be an overarching elegant theory that explains the constellation of symptoms.

Research method of this report: In arriving at this theory, the analysis is not restricted in any particular health field and all sources of relevant information is included as best as possible (i.e. scientific reports, academic texts, health reviews, personal testimonials, observation of the author's own family challenges etc.). Nonetheless, the missing gaps to connect the silos are based on the author's own theorization. Assumptions underlying this report are that amidst the myriad of symptoms, there is intelligence in the body and an order to things.

Disclaimer: The author of this report is not trained in the health field. However, perhaps because of this, there is an advantage to relook at the problem and solutions from an entirely unbiased new perspective. Nonetheless, the author's skillset as a risk manager (i.e. probing experts in their fields to list problem statements, close the gaps/silos, find the root causes to problems and mitigating actions) applied in these particular health challenges of personal interest as many in the author's family were afflicted with either metabolic syndrome or mental health challenges, underpinned the passion to understand the real root cause for these disorders, and to find a natural solution to long lasting healing.

Use this report with caution.

Nonetheless, do use this report as a guide for your own research and advocacy.

The radical theory on MetS and Depression proposed here will:

1) Present the real reasons and symptoms for MetS and distinguish between lean MetS vs. overweight MetS along the MetS spectrum.

2) This proposed theory would also demonstrate that Borderline Personality Disorder (BPD) is in fact a type of depression, which borders between normalcy and extreme emotions (Borderline depression). Additionally, this report will show how BPD/Borderline depression is interrelated with MetS.

3) Present the real reasons and symptoms for depression and distinguish between Dysthymia, BPD/Borderline depression, Bipolar depression and Major depression along the mania-depression spectrum.

4) Highlight the key factors connecting between MetS and depression, and demonstrate the different combination manifestations of these 2 disorders (i.e. MetS with BPD/Borderline depression, MetS with Dysthymia, MetS with Bipolar and MetS with Major depression & anxiety).

5) Crucially, this report will demonstrate that these 2 seemingly disparate but interrelated disorders (i.e. MetS and depression) are due to overexertion of our body (i.e. physical and/or mental) in countering a stress and that the overexertion can be reversed through the right nutrition (expedited with the aid of a mere 4 supplements) and right mental coping. Hence, *there is hope for healing*!

(A) Stress and its relationship with energy levels

(i) Energy intake

The body just needs the optimal nutrient and calorie or energy intake level for its activities. However, in times of chronic stress, the body certainly requires more energy but just enough to meet its needs. Unfortunately, many of us lack the correct nutritional knowledge, and our energy intake becomes either higher or lower than required. For example;

- When the body's intake of glucose becomes too high and the liver/pancreas is overworked, we have *insulin resistance* [refer section D(i-1)]. Conversely, when it's too low, we have anxiety and trembling (hunger for food to replenish the depleting energy level), refer C(ii-4).

- Lower protein intake makes it *harder for the body to replenish hormones and neurotransmitters* as protein is the building block for them. Also, chronic stress can catabolise protein stores in our body's muscles to fuel the immediate energy requirement, thus, *our metabolism slows down with loss of muscle tone* which leads to a higher potential for more glucose & fat storage (*obesity*), refer C(ii-1), C(ii-2) and C(ii-3). Depleted protein from our gut muscle will lead to *leaky gut and an impaired immunity* (autoimmune/ allergies) [refer section C(ii-5) and C(ii-6)].

- If our fat intake is too high, there is potential for obesity and *acne* [refer C(ii-3)], and if our intake of essential fatty acid is too *low, our cell membrane health is adversely affected* (refer section B).

- Inadequate vitamins/minerals and antioxidants would *impair our methylation process*, leading to various issues as stated in section C(i). Importantly, a weak methylation status makes us *susceptible to major illnesses* (i.e. MetS, BPD, major depression) because the body easily succumbs to the effects of chronic stress (refer section C figure C(i)1).

The optimal nutrient intake will prepare our body to withstand stress when it arises. Else, stress will magnify our pre-existing body imbalances.

(ii) Energy redirection and amplification of mental resilience & intimidating physical features

During the cavemen days, a stress denotes a threat to life. During a threat/stress, the body adapted through suppressing sex hormones production by the sex gland and using the same base ingredient (pregnenolone) in favour of cortisol production by the adrenal gland [refer section D(ii), which talks about the 'cortisol steal'] to fight/flee and *prioritising survival over fertility* [refer section D(ii), where fertility is suppressed]. The liver which produces cholesterol (a precursor to pregnenolone) has to overwork to ensure the needs of both the sex and adrenal glands are met.

To conserve energy to fight/flee, the body slows down the digestion of fats as they require more time, effort and resources by slowing down bile production from the liver to the stomach. Hence, *digestion* [refer section D(iv)] is suppressed.

Additionally, there will be protein catabolisation at the muscles to supply immediate energy for quick reflex actions. Hence, protein depletion will impair *metabolism* [refer section C(ii-1)] and *growth, healing & immunity* [refer section C(ii-6) where Arginine, a protein crucial for immune and wound/tissue repairs, is depleted during times of stress. Additionally, Glutamine is also depleted during times of stress. Glutamine is a protein which prevents leaky gut (note: leaky gut leads to autoimmunity issues and a loss of nutrient absorption) and as well as being a precursor to Glutathione, which is a master antioxidant that serves as a defence/protection against free radical damages].

The body's cholesterol profile will become weak due to the slowdown of the body's *circulatory* function [refer section D(iii)], an unfortunate consequence of prioritising immediate survivability.

In our modern times, not all forms of stress construe to a threat. Hence, a sad feeling over an incident is not a threat, hence, the body will not redirect energy to activate cortisol. Mainly, *a stress that makes us fearful/anxious* (or low GABA, refer to section F(ii) for information on neurotransmitters spectrum of emotions & functions) *activates cortisol, and the body redirects its resources to support cortisol activation* [refer section D(ii)].

Apart from the above redirection of energy usage, there will be amplification of energy where;

- the *physical features become more masculine and intimidating* to ward of threats:
  This is triggered by *5 alpha reductase*, an enzyme that amplifies the conversion of testosterone to **DHT**, a more powerful androgen with effects on the central nervous system, skin/face and hair scalp. The skin/face will have more pronounced masculine features such as thicker moustache or beard and severe acne. 5 alpha reductase is a biomarker for MetS.

- the *mind becomes more focused and driven* to handle the threat/stress:
  With regards to the effects on the central nervous system, a *metabolite of DHT called 3b-adiol stimulates only the estrogen receptor beta (ERβ) in the brain* (Link 7). ERβ is associated with *signalling of oxytocinergic neurons to produce oxytocin* (by the pituitary gland) (Link 8). *Oxytocin enhances activity in dopaminergic regions* and animal studies have shown the existence of numerous oxytocin receptors throughout the dopamine system (Link 9). *Oxytocin enhances glutamate activity* (Link 10).

  The reason for the increase of oxytocin, dopamine and glutamate levels in the brain is so that *the body becomes more focused (high oxytocin), more perceptive (high glutamate) and more driven to act (high dopamine)* to counter the threat. Additionally, *higher activation of ERβ [instead of its opposing estrogen receptor alpha (ERα)] will increase serotonin (ease/comfort) and increase GABA (calmness or less anxiety),* refer (Link 11). Feeling at ease and calm in countering a threat is an important survival instinct.

  Note 1: Refer to section F(ii) for information on neurotransmitters (brain chemicals) spectrum of emotions & functions i.e. oxytocin, dopamine, glutamate, serotonin, GABA.

  Note 2: ERα is highly expressed in the liver while ERβ is highly expressed in the brain. Refer to (Link 11), an article about functions and physiological roles of the two types of estrogen receptors, ERα and ERβ, identified by estrogen knockout mouse.

  Note 3: ERβ activation enhances oxytocin level which then enhances prolactin level. High prolactin level will suppress fertility.

Multiple studies have demonstrated that the activation of estrogen receptors (ERα and ERβ) can influence hypothalamic-pituitary-adrenal (HPA) responses to stress, (refer Link 12). *Selective activation of ERα can amplify (or exaggerate) HPA reactivity to stress, whereas selective activation of ERβ can reduce the reactivity (or exaggeration) of the HPA axis to stressors* (Link 13).

Males also express estrogen receptors (ERs) in the liver as they serve important metabolic functions in males. For example, the aromatization (i.e. transformation) of testosterone to estradiol (i.e. a form of estrogen) is beneficial for preventing central obesity in men. ERα is the predominant ER subtype in both male and female hepatocytes (liver cells), (Link 14).

Aromatization

❖ At the sex gland, testosterone is either aromatised (via the aromatase enzyme) to estradiol (i.e. a form of estrogen) and bind to estrogen receptor (ER) or converted to DHT (via 5 alpha reductase enzyme) and bind to androgen receptor (AR), (Link 14).

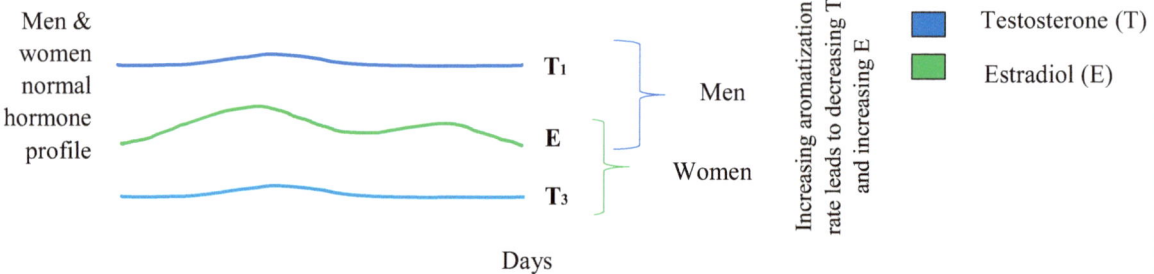

Figure A1: Aromatization rate which impacts the gender normal hormone profile (i.e. Men has $T_1 > E$ while women has $E > T_3$)

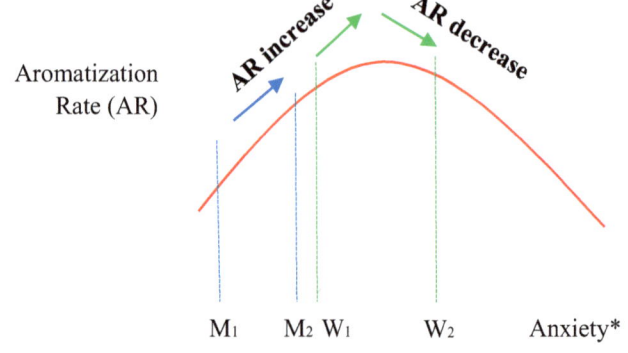

Figure A2: Comparison of AR between Men (M) and Women (W)

The starting aromatization rate (AR) for men is lower than women's (i.e. $M_1 < W_1$).

The women's AR at position W_1 is almost reaching the peak of the AR/Anxiety bell curve.

Due to the above, chronic anxiety or anxious type of stress for men will result in AR increases while for women, depending on the chronic level of the anxiety, will lead to AR increases and eventually decreases.

* Anxiety (or low GABA) triggers [recap from A(ii)]:
- Physical pathway: Cortisol hormone increment → Cortisol steal → Sex hormone depletion → Overworking of liver [in particular, estrogen receptor alpha (ERα) at the liver] to balance cortisol vs sex hormone level, produced by the adrenal and sex gland respectively [In summary, anxious stress overworks the liver/adrenal/sex gland, adversely impacting our metabolic/ endocrine health]

- Mental pathway: 5 alpha reductase activation → DHT activation → 3b-adiol activation → over activation of estrogen receptor beta (ERβ) in the brain → high oxytocin level (i.e. brain excitability) → high prolactin level (i.e. fertility suppression) [In summary, anxious stress leads to higher brain excitability and suppresses our fertility]

Aromatization rate (AR)	20%	40%	60%	80%	100%
Testosterone (T_1)	100	100	100	100	100
Estradiol (E)	20	40	60	80	100
Testosterone (T_2)	80	60	40	20	0

Figure A3: Relationship between AR, Testosterone and Estradiol. (When AR increases, T_2 decreases while E increases. Conversely, when AR decreases, T_2 increases while E decreases)

Scenario 1: Aromatization rate increase (therefore, decreasing T and increasing E)
- ❖ The aromatization rate can be increased due to metabolic syndrome (MetS) factors or endocrine issues such as obesity, insulin resistance, inflammation and consumption of alcohol, [(Link 15) and (Link 16)].
- ❖ For men, increasing aromatization rate will lead to decreasing T with increasing E, resulting in the feminization of men.
- ❖ For women, increasing aromatization rate will lead to decreasing T with increasing E, resulting in estrogen dominance in women.

Scenario 2: Aromatization rate decrease (therefore, increasing T and decreasing E)
- ❖ The aromatization rate can be decreased by prolactin (note: a high level of anxiety will increase prolactin level) and anti-Mullerian hormone, [(Link 15) and (Link 16)].
- ❖ Decreasing aromatization rate will lead to increasing T with decreasing E, resulting in excessive androgen level, which can cause severe acne in both male and female.
- ❖ Increased testosterone or hyperandrogenism in men is associated with more aggression in men.
- ❖ Increased testosterone or hyperandrogenism in women is associated with PCOS or the masculinization of women, (Link 14).

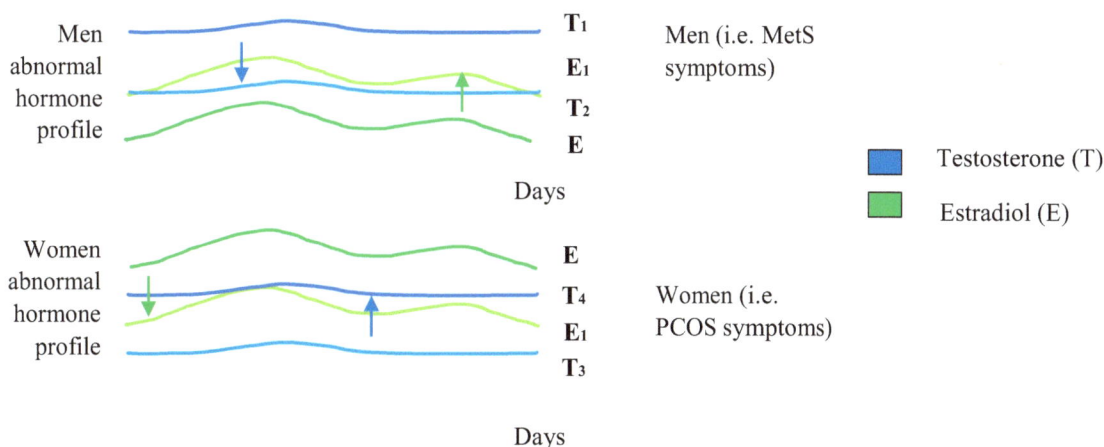

Figure A4: Chronic anxiety affecting the aromatization rate, which leads to the gender abnormal hormonal profile (i.e. Men has $T_2 < E_1$ while women has $E_1 < T_4$). Abnormal hormonal profile is associated with metabolic/endocrine problems for men (i.e. MetS) and women (i.e. PCOS)

Scenario 3: Weakened liver and sex gland due to chronic anxiety (therefore, low T and low E)
- ❖ Chronic anxious stress will at first cause the aromatization rate at the sex gland to increase and when the sex gland reaches a fatigue point, the aromatization rate will decrease, thus, leading to increasing testosterone (T) and decreasing estrogen (E). However, if the sex gland becomes too fatigue, even T will eventually decrease, and we will then have a situation of both low T and low E for both men and women.
- ❖ Decreasing estrogen would then result in spontaneous obesity in both male and female, (Link 14).
- ❖ Low estrogen promotes fat deposition in the liver. Hence, estrogen is important in both male and female in the regulation of lipogenesis in the liver, (Link 14).

Figure A5: Relationship between aromatization, testosterone & estrogen level, androgen & estrogen receptor

The next pages in figures A(ii)1, A(iii)1, A(iii)2, A(iii)3, A(iii)4 and A(iii)5 will demonstrate the concepts discussed here.

In short, chronic anxious stress will trigger our body into a survival mode, redirecting the body's energy in favour for survival over fertility, digestion, metabolism, circulatory, growth, healing & immunity. Chronic anxious stress will also prioritize survival over our attractiveness and long term physical & mental health.

Radical theory on MetS & Depression

```
                        Testosterone  ──→  DHT & its metabolite
              aromatase      │        5 alpha reductase      │
                             ▼                                ▼
Estrogen receptor alpha (ERα) ←── Estradiol ──→ Estrogen receptor beta (ERβ)
```

5 alpha reductase=0 because no anxiety, Normal aromatization rate	Normal aromatization of testosterone to estradiol
DHT	No DHT
Testosterone (T)	Baseline level
Estradiol (E)	Baseline level
ERβ to ERα activation ratio	ERβ/ERα=1 because only estradiol acts in equal amount on ERβ & ERα
Mood balancing to counter stress (i.e. survival instinct) (higher ERβ activation, the more serotonin & GABA while higher ERα activation, the less serotonin & GABA)	At ease and calm
Fertility	Good because body is not under anxiety and no higher ERβ activation

5 alpha reductase increases due to anxiety trigger, Aromatization rate increases	Greater aromatization of testosterone to estradiol
DHT	DHT amplified from testosterone (i.e. androgenic)
Testosterone (T)	Reduce from baseline level due to increased aromatization and cortisol steal
Estradiol (E)	Increase from baseline due to increased aromatization but at a slow rate due to cortisol steal
ERβ to ERα activation ratio	ERβ/ERα>1 because both estradiol & DHT metabolite act on ERβ while only estradiol acts on ERα
Mood balancing to counter stress (i.e. survival instinct) (higher ERβ activation, the more serotonin & GABA while higher ERα activation, the less serotonin & GABA)	High serotonin and high GABA (highly at ease and highly calm)
Fertility	Reduced fertility due to higher ERβ activation

Figure A(ii)1: Impact of 5 alpha reductase and aromatization rate on DHT, Testosterone, Estradiol, ERα, ERβ, mood balancing and fertility

Note: Refer to You Tube video at The Fruitful Society entitled – [Basics to "A radical theory on men metabolic syndrome/ infertility (MetS) & Depression"] for numerical application of the above.

(iii) *Over exertion of energy countered by nutritional & mental coping methods*

However, chronic prolonged stress will over exert our energy level and this will impact us both physically and mentally. How we cope will determine whether we manifest MetS or Borderline depression/Borderline Personality Disorder (BPD) or Dysthymia or Bipolar or Major depression with anxiety.

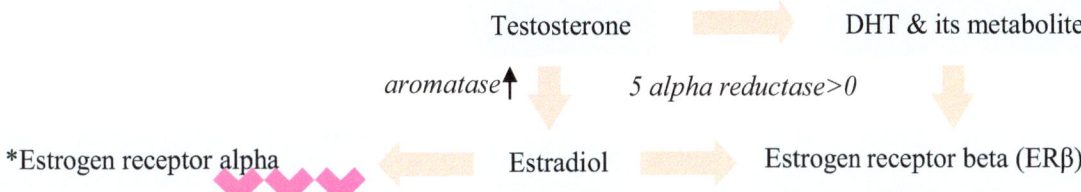

*Extremely overexerted liver results in excessive free radical damages on ERα at liver

5 alpha reductase increases due to anxiety trigger, Aromatization rate increases	Extreme aromatization of testosterone to estradiol
DHT	More DHT amplified from testosterone (i.e. androgenic, acne at chin area)
Testosterone (T)	Reduce from baseline due to increased aromatization & cortisol steal
Estradiol (E)	Increase from baseline due to increased aromatization but at a slow rate due to cortisol steal
ERβ to ERα activation ratio	ERβ/ERα ratio is extremely high as ERα is damaged and thus, more estradiol acts on ERβ alongside with more DHT metabolite that act on ERβ
Mood balancing to counter stress (i.e. survival instinct) (higher ERβ activation, the more serotonin & GABA while higher ERα activation, the less serotonin & GABA)	Extremely high serotonin and extremely high GABA (extremely at ease and extremely calm)
Fertility	Extremely high ERβ activation due to anxiety means extremely high oxytocin by the pituitary gland leading to extremely high prolactin which results in infertility

Figure A(iii)1: Wrong coping to support the extremely overexerted liver during extreme anxious stress results in MetS

Note: Refer to You Tube video at The Fruitful Society entitled – [Basics to "A radical theory on men metabolic syndrome/ infertility (MetS) & Depression"] for numerical application of the above.

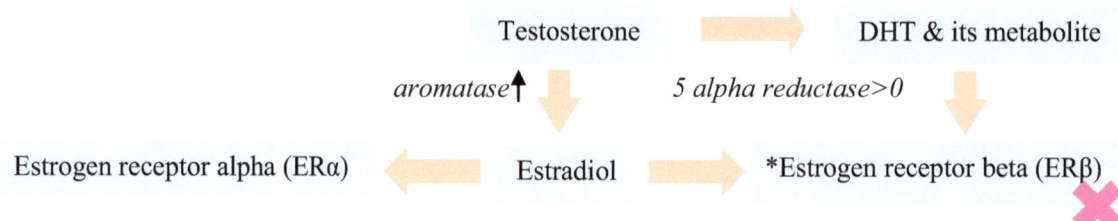

Low overexerted brain results in low free radical damages on ERβ at the brain

5 alpha reductase increases due to anxiety trigger, Aromatization rate increases	Normal aromatization rate	Increased aromatization rate (hence declining T and increasing E)
DHT	DHT amplified from testosterone (i.e. androgenic)	More DHT amplified from testosterone (i.e. androgenic, acne at forehead)
Testosterone (T)	Reduce from baseline due to increased aromatization & cortisol steal	Reduce from baseline due to increased aromatization & cortisol steal
Estradiol (E)	Increase from baseline due to increased aromatization but at a slow rate due to cortisol steal	Increase from baseline due to increased aromatization but at a slow rate due to cortisol steal
ERβ to ERα activation ratio	ERβ/ERα>1 because both estradiol & DHT metabolite act on ERβ while only estradiol acts on ERα	ERβ/ERα<1. With some ERβ being damaged, DHT metabolite acts on ERβ while increasing estradiol redirects to act on ERα
Mood balancing to counter stress (i.e. survival instinct) (higher ERβ activation, the more serotonin & GABA while higher ERα activation, the less serotonin & GABA)	High serotonin and high GABA (highly at ease and highly calm)	Slightly low serotonin and slightly low GABA (slightly frustrated and slightly anxious)
Fertility	Reduced fertility as higher ERβ activation due to anxiety means higher oxytocin by the pituitary gland leading to higher prolactin. High level of prolactin suppresses fertility	Reduced fertility as higher ERβ activation due to anxiety means higher oxytocin by the pituitary gland leading to higher prolactin. High level of prolactin suppresses fertility

Figure A(iii)2: Wrong coping in supporting the low overexerted brain during times of low emotional stress results in Borderline Personality Disorder or Borderline depression symptoms

Note: Refer to You Tube video at The Fruitful Society entitled – [Basics to "A radical theory on men metabolic syndrome/ infertility (MetS) & Depression"] for numerical application of the above.

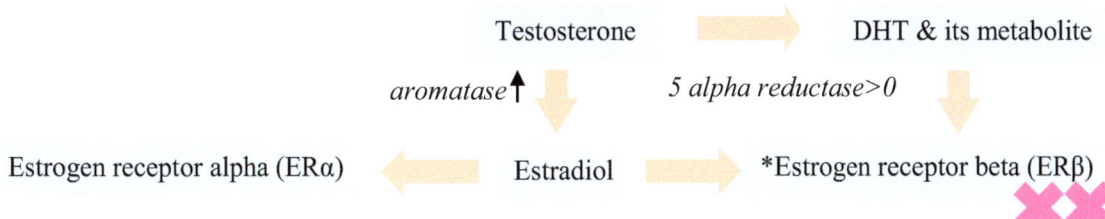

Moderately overexerted brain results in a moderate number of free radical damages on ERβ at the brain

5 alpha reductase increases due to anxiety trigger, Aromatization rate increases	Normal aromatization rate	Increased aromatization rate (hence declining T and increasing E)
DHT	DHT amplified from testosterone (i.e. androgenic)	More DHT amplified from testosterone (i.e. androgenic, acne at forehead)
Testosterone (T)	Reduce from baseline due to increased aromatization & cortisol steal	Reduce from baseline due to increased aromatization & cortisol steal
Estradiol (E)	Increase from baseline due to increased aromatization but at a slow rate due to cortisol steal	Increase from baseline due to increased aromatization but at a slow rate due to cortisol steal
ERβ to ERα activation ratio	ERβ/ERα<1 because with more ERβ being damaged, DHT metabolite acts on ERβ while estradiol redirects to act on ERα	ERβ/ERα<<1. With more ERβ being damaged, DHT metabolite acts on ERβ while increasing estradiol redirects to act on ERα
Mood balancing to counter stress (i.e. survival instinct) (higher ERβ activation, the more serotonin & GABA while higher ERα activation, the less serotonin & GABA)	Slightly low serotonin and slightly low GABA (slightly frustrated and slightly anxious)	Low serotonin and low GABA (frustrated and anxious)
Fertility	Reduced fertility as higher ERβ activation due to anxiety means higher oxytocin by the pituitary gland leading to higher prolactin. High level of prolactin suppresses fertility	Reduced fertility as higher ERβ activation due to anxiety means higher oxytocin by the pituitary gland leading to higher prolactin. High level of prolactin suppresses fertility

Figure A(iii)3: Wrong coping in supporting the moderately overexerted brain during times of moderate emotional stress results in Dysthymia symptoms

Note: Refer to You Tube video at The Fruitful Society entitled – [Basics to "A radical theory on men metabolic syndrome/ infertility (MetS) & Depression"] for numerical application of the above.

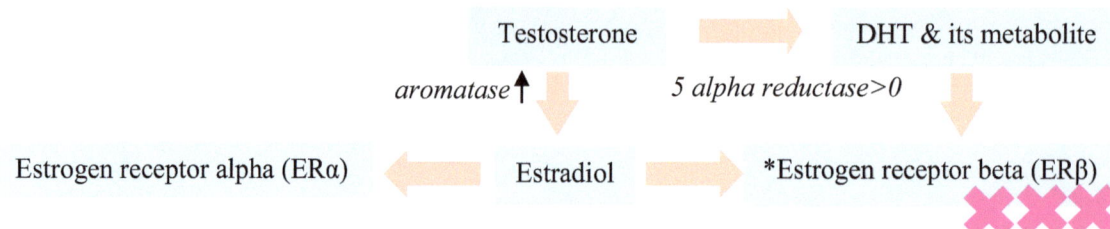

Highly overexerted brain results in a high number of free radical damages on ERβ at the brain

5 alpha reductase increases due to anxiety trigger, Aromatization rate increases	Normal aromatization rate	Increased aromatization rate (hence declining T and increasing E)
DHT	DHT amplified from testosterone (i.e. androgenic)	More DHT amplified from testosterone (i.e. androgenic, acne at forehead)
Testosterone (T)	Reduce from baseline due to increased aromatization & cortisol steal	Reduce from baseline due to increased aromatization & cortisol steal
Estradiol (E)	Increase from baseline due to increased aromatization but at a slow rate due to cortisol steal	Increase from baseline due to increased aromatization but at a slow rate due to cortisol steal
ERβ to ERα activation ratio	ERβ/ERα<<1 because with even more ERβ being damaged, DHT metabolite acts on ERβ while estradiol redirects to act on ERα	ERβ/ERα<<<1. With even more ERβ being damaged, DHT metabolite acts on ERβ while increasing estradiol redirects to act on ERα
Mood balancing to counter stress (i.e. survival instinct) (higher ERβ activation, the more serotonin & GABA while higher ERα activation, the less serotonin & GABA)	Low serotonin and low GABA (frustrated and anxious)	Very low serotonin and very low GABA (very frustrated and very anxious)
Fertility	Reduced fertility as higher ERβ activation due to anxiety means higher oxytocin by the pituitary gland leading to higher prolactin. High level of prolactin suppresses fertility	Reduced fertility as higher ERβ activation due to anxiety means higher oxytocin by the pituitary gland leading to higher prolactin. High level of prolactin suppresses fertility

Figure A(iii)4: Wrong coping in supporting the highly overexerted brain during times of moderate emotional stress results in Bipolar symptoms

Note 1:
- Bipolar I   : Consists of mania – moderate/major depression phase
- Bipolar II   : Consists of hypomania – moderate/major depression phase

Note: Refer to You Tube video at The Fruitful Society entitled – [Basics to "A radical theory on men metabolic syndrome/ infertility (MetS) & Depression"] for numerical application of the above.

Radical theory on MetS & Depression

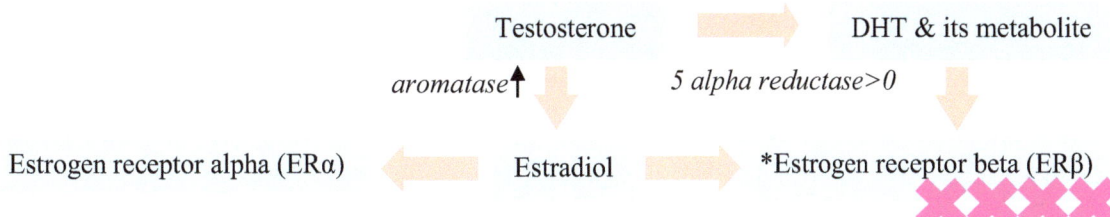

Extremely overexerted brain results in excessive free radical damages on ERβ at the brain

5 alpha reductase increases due to anxiety trigger, Aromatization rate increases	Normal aromatization rate	Increased aromatization rate (hence declining T and increasing E)
DHT	DHT amplified from testosterone (i.e. androgenic)	More DHT amplified from testosterone (i.e. androgenic, acne at forehead)
Testosterone (T)	Reduce from baseline due to increased aromatization & cortisol steal	Reduce from baseline due to increased aromatization & cortisol steal
Estradiol (E)	Increase from baseline due to increased aromatization but at a slow rate due to cortisol steal	Increase from baseline due to increased aromatization but at a slow rate due to cortisol steal
ERβ to ERα activation ratio	ERβ/ERα<<<1 because with a large proportion of ERβ being damaged, DHT metabolite acts on ERβ while estradiol redirects to act on ERα	ERβ/ERα<<<<1. With a large proportion of ERβ being damaged, DHT metabolite acts on ERβ while increasing estradiol redirects to act on ERα
Mood balancing to counter stress (i.e. survival instinct) (higher ERβ activation, the more serotonin & GABA while higher ERα activation, the less serotonin & GABA)	Very low serotonin and very low GABA (very frustrated and very anxious)	Extremely low serotonin and extremely low GABA (extremely frustrated and extremely anxious)
Fertility	Reduced fertility as higher ERβ activation due to anxiety means higher oxytocin by the pituitary gland leading to higher prolactin. High level of prolactin suppresses fertility	Reduced fertility as higher ERβ activation due to anxiety means higher oxytocin by the pituitary gland leading to higher prolactin. High level of prolactin suppresses fertility

Figure A(iii)5: Wrong coping in supporting the extremely overexerted brain during times of extreme emotional stress results in Major depression with anxiety

Note: Refer to You Tube video at The Fruitful Society entitled – [Basics to "A radical theory on men metabolic syndrome/ infertility (MetS) & Depression"] for numerical application of the above.

It is interesting to note that Chinese face mapping says that acne at chin area denotes a hormonal imbalance with excess androgen (relates to the liver as per figure A(iii)1) while acne at forehead denotes mental stress (relates to the brain as per figure A(iii)2, A(iii)3, A(iii)4 and A(iii)5). Refer to (Link 17).

Depression type	Free radical damage on ERβ at brain	Mental over exertion	ERβ to ERα activation ratio, which indicates the mood balancing to counter anxious stress (i.e. survival instinct)	
			Normal aromatization rate	Increased aromatization rate (hence declining T and increasing E)
Nil (Mentally healthy)	Nil	Nil	ERβ/ERα>1	ERβ/ERα>1
			High serotonin & high GABA (highly at ease & highly calm)	High serotonin & high GABA (highly at ease & highly calm)
Borderline/ BPD	Low	Low	ERβ/ERα>1	ERβ/ERα<1
			High serotonin & high GABA (highly at ease & highly calm)	Slightly low serotonin & slightly low GABA (slightly frustrated & slightly anxious)
Dysthymia	Moderate	Moderate	ERβ/ERα<1	ERβ/ERα<<1
			Slightly low serotonin & slightly low GABA (slightly frustrated & slightly anxious)	Low serotonin & low GABA (frustrated & anxious)
Bipolar II	High	High	ERβ/ERα<<1	ERβ/ERα<<<1
			Low serotonin & low GABA (frustrated & anxious)	Very low serotonin & very low GABA (very frustrated & very anxious)
	Moderately excessive protein intake level [refer figure A(iii)8]		Baseline serotonin & low GABA (at ease & anxious)	Low serotonin & very low GABA (frustrated & very anxious)
Major	Extreme	Extreme	ERβ/ERα<<<1	ERβ/ERα<<<<1
			Very low serotonin & very low GABA (very frustrated & very anxious)	Extremely low serotonin & extremely low GABA (extremely frustrated & extremely anxious)

(Stress coping: Good → Bad)

Figure A(iii)6: Comparison of mood fluctuations within differing aromatization rate between Borderline depression/ BPD, Dysthymia, Bipolar II and Major depression based on figure A(iii)2/ 3/ 4/ 5 respectively

Summary analysis of figure A(iii)6:
- Stress coping deteriorates when there are more free radical damages on ERβ at the brain.
- Estrogen fluctuations impact the mood.
- Mood worsens when there are more testosterone being aromatised to estrogen due to MetS factors. The *estrogen increases* cause the ERβ/ERα ratio to be less than 1, where the ratio is impacted by *the degree of damaged ERβ*.
- The more free radical damages on ERβ at the brain, the smaller the ERβ/ERα ratio because estrogen increases would then be redirected to activate ERα instead of ERβ.
- The smaller the ERβ/ERα ratio, the lower the serotonin level (i.e. denoting frustration) and the lower the GABA level (i.e. denoting anxiety). Conversely, the higher the ERβ/ERα ratio, the higher the serotonin level (i.e. denoting feeling at ease) and the higher the GABA level (i.e. denoting calmness).
- According to the National Institute of Mental Health (NIMH) of America, women are 70% more likely than men to experience depression during their lifetime. This is due to women having more estrogen fluctuations as part of their menstrual cycle which impact the mood.

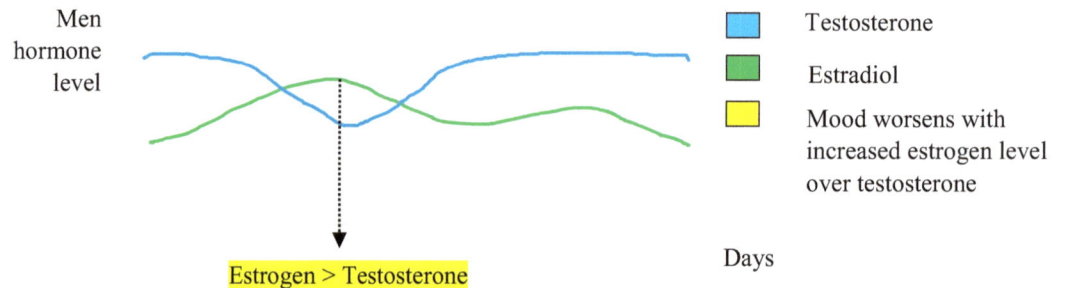

Figure A(iii)7: Increased estrogen level can be associated with depression in men (Link 18)

	Mania Spectrum			Depression Spectrum			
	Bipolar I	**Bipolar II**	**Borderline**	**Borderline**	**Dysthymia**	**Bipolar I & Bipolar II**	**Major**
Emotional stress	Extreme	Moderate	Baseline	Low	Moderate	Moderate	Extreme
Wrong mental coping: (i.e. Rumination)	Extreme	Moderate	Baseline	Low	Moderate	Moderate	Extreme
Wrong nutrient coping: (i.e. Excessive protein)	Extreme	Moderate					
Mental overexertion	Extreme	High	Baseline	Low	Moderate	High	Extreme

Figure A(iii)8: Key differences between Borderline depression, Dysthymia depression, Bipolar and Major depression along the mania-depression spectrum

Summary analysis of figure A(iii)8:
- Mood disorders can be quantified along the mania-depression spectrum.
- Oftentimes, there are misdiagnoses due to the interchangeability of the mood disorder along the spectrum.
- The items highlighted in blue are the factors contributing toward the mood disorders.
- The item highlighted in orange denotes the degree of mental overexertion.
- For instance:
    - Borderline depression/BPD fluctuates between baseline normal of the mania-depression spectrum and at the low end of the depression spectrum, where the factors contributing to it are low emotional stress and low wrong mental coping leading to a low mental overexertion.
    - Dysthymia is at the moderate end of the depression spectrum, where the factors contributing to it are moderate emotional stress and moderate wrong mental coping leading to a moderate mental overexertion.
    - Bipolar II fluctuates between high end of the mania spectrum (i.e. hypomania) and high-extreme end of the depression spectrum, where the factors contributing to it are moderate emotional stress, moderate wrong mental coping and a moderate excessive protein level intake leading to a high mental overexertion.
    - Bipolar I fluctuates between extreme end of the mania spectrum and high-extreme end of the depression spectrum, where the factors contributing to it are extreme emotional stress, extreme wrong mental coping and an extreme excessive protein level intake leading to an extreme mental overexertion.
    - Major depression is at the extreme end of the depression spectrum, where the factors contributing to it are extreme emotional stress and extreme wrong mental coping leading to an extreme mental overexertion.

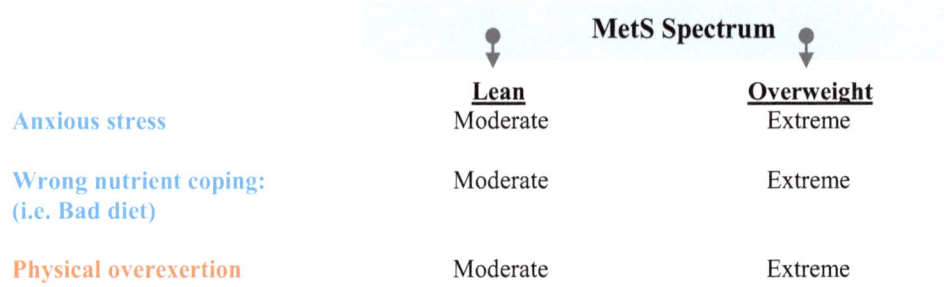

Figure A(iii)9: Key differences between Lean and Overweight MetS along the MetS spectrum

Summary analysis of figure A(iii)9:
- MetS can be quantified along the MetS spectrum.
- The items highlighted in blue are the factors contributing toward the MetS.
- The item highlighted in orange denotes the degree of physical overexertion.
- For instance:
    - MetS (lean type) is at the moderate end of the MetS spectrum, where the factors contributing to it are moderate anxious stress and moderate wrong nutrient coping leading to a moderate physical overexertion.
    - MetS (overweight type) is at the extreme end of the MetS spectrum, where the factors contributing to it are extreme anxious stress and extreme wrong nutrient coping leading to an extreme physical overexertion.

Based on the concepts explored thus far, the key differentiation between manifestations of MetS only symptoms; BPD/Borderline depression only symptoms; Dysthymia only symptoms; Bipolar only symptoms; Major depression with anxiety only symptoms; MetS with BPD/Borderline depression symptoms; MetS with Dysthymia symptoms; MetS with Bipolar symptoms; MetS with Major depression and anxiety symptoms are as follows:

- The energy intake during the stressful period:
    - Whether high or low or adequate diet intake for each nutrient type (i.e. protein/ carbohydrate/ fats/ vitamins/ minerals/ antioxidant).
    - A low intake of protein/ high intake of simple carbohydrate/ high intake of bad fats will predispose the body towards a metabolic/ endocrine problem.
    - Meanwhile, a low intake of vitamins/ minerals/ antioxidants will predispose the body towards a methylation problem.

- The context of the stress:
    - Whether does it instil worry/anxiousness/fear? If yes, energy redirection and energy amplification by the body (both physically and mentally) will take place because the body thinks it is facing a threat for survival.

- The coping style (how we respond to the stressor) to prevent over exertion:
    - Further physical or nutritional wrong coping method will lead to metabolic syndrome/ infertility problems.
    - Further mental wrong coping method will lead to mental health/ depression [i.e. borderline depression (BPD), dysthymia, bipolar or major depression with anxiety] problems.

Note: The following case studies item (iv) – (xvii) will further demonstrate the concepts above.

(iv) Metabolic Syndrome (MetS) case study

Variables	Example	Body mechanism	Reference section
Energy (diet) intake	Diet of high simple glucose, high bad fat, low protein, low vitamins, low minerals and low antioxidant	Low protein: predisposition to endocrine/metabolic issues	C(ii-1) – metabolism D(i) – metabolic issues
		High simple glucose: predisposition to endocrine/metabolic issues, high free radicals	C(ii-2) – excess glucose D(i) – metabolic issues B – free radical
		Excess bad fat: predisposition to endocrine/metabolic issues	C(ii-3) – fats D(i) – metabolic issues
		Low vitamins/minerals/antioxidant with *gene problems* (**MTHFR**/MTRR/COMT/MAO-A): *predisposition to methylation issues*	C(i) – methylation
Context & timing of the stress which determine energy redirection & amplification	Extreme anxiety (low GABA) to achieve work deadlines overworks the liver	Trigger of energy redirection due to anxiety, hence, predisposition to endocrine/metabolic issue via: • *Cortisol steal*: suppressing sex hormones production in favour of cortisol production • *Conservation of energy*: through slow down digestion of fats • *Catabolisation of protein*: to supply immediate energy for reflex action, depleting our body's protein	A(ii) D(ii) D(iv) C(ii-1)
		Trigger of energy amplification due to anxiety, measured by an *increase in 5 alpha reductase*. *Androgenic* with amplification on both physical and mental traits	A(ii)
Coping style to prevent over exertion	Extreme bad diet: Low protein, bad fats and high glucose intake unable to support liver functions in stress handling Also, low vitamins/minerals/ antioxidants predispose to methylation impairment	*Extreme overexertion* of the liver to support extreme anxious stress handling. Overworked liver has higher vibration attracting free radical attacks. *Methylation gene defect expression* will cause *antioxidant defence against free radical damages to be low*, leading to *extreme free radical damage* at the liver (ERα) and triggering *inflammation, oxidative stress* & liver *insulin resistance*. Thus, *water/nutrients/oxygen cannot be properly absorbed into liver cells*, impairing liver's *hydroxylation* process. Liver weakens resulting in a hormonal imbalance (which *cannot be restored to baseline levels due to methylation and oxygen deprivation problems*) thus leading to MetS, infertility. Refer item (v) below for all associated symptoms	B – free radical attack C(i) – methylation A Figure A(iii)1 –free radical damage at liver D – impact of free radical damage on neuroendocrine

Figure A(iv)1: MetS case study: How nutrition, gene predisposition, and stress coping leads to or prevents MetS

Note: MetS shares the same key root cause (highlighted in orange above) and impaired body mechanism (highlighted in purple above) with BPD/Borderline depression (figure A(vi)1), Dysthymia (figure A(viii)1), Bipolar (figure A(x)1) and Major depression with anxiety (figure A(xii)1).

(v) *MetS symptoms & root causes*

<table>
<tr><th>Symptoms</th><th>Root cause</th><th>Reference section</th></tr>
<tr><td rowspan="11">**Noticeable symptoms**</td><td></td><td></td></tr>
<tr><td>Severe acne</td><td>High cholesterol and fat level (elevated lipids), decreasing antioxidant status, increasing DHT along with a weak immune (arising from low levels of vitamin A & D) to combat acne bacteria</td><td>D(i-5) – acne
D(iii) – cholesterol
D(i-1) – fats
C – antioxidant
A(ii) – DHT
D(iv) – vitamin A & D</td></tr>
<tr><td>Blur vision</td><td>Low levels of vitamin A</td><td>D(iv)</td></tr>
<tr><td>Skin issues (i.e. rashes, bruising)</td><td>Bile sluggishness and low levels of vitamin E & K</td><td>D(iv)</td></tr>
<tr><td>Reduced skin vibrancy</td><td>Lower glutamine to make collagen</td><td>C(ii-1) – glutamine</td></tr>
<tr><td>**Central obesity (i.e. high triglycerides)**</td><td>Weakened liver unable to store excess glucose as glycogen in the liver but redirected to fat cells combined with a low estrogen status</td><td>D(i-1) – triglycerides
D(i-4) – central obesity
D(ii) – hormones</td></tr>
<tr><td>Gut issues (i.e. constipation, bloating)</td><td>Bile sluggishness arising from a weak liver</td><td>D(iv)</td></tr>
<tr><td>Easily get infections/ weak immunity</td><td>Weakened immunity (due to low levels of vitamin A & D)</td><td>D(iv)</td></tr>
<tr><td>Knee pain</td><td>Lowered glucosamine in knee joints arising from lower glutamine</td><td>C(ii-1) – glutamine</td></tr>
<tr><td>Higher likelihood of anxiety, depression, BPD and other mental health issues</td><td>Negative mental coping (i.e. mental stress over adverse MetS symptoms listed here or other life's stresses)</td><td>F, G, H</td></tr>
<tr><td>Feminization (i.e. breast tissue growth)</td><td>Decreasing testosterone level and increasing estrogen level due to aromatization triggered by metabolic syndrome (Link 19)</td><td>D(ii)</td></tr>
<tr><td>Fertility issues, sexual dysfunction</td><td>Hormonal imbalance</td><td>D(ii)</td></tr>
</table>

Symptoms	Root cause	Reference section
Sperm problems, low sex drive	Low vitamin D, low sex hormones	D(iv) and D(ii) – vitamin D D(ii) – hormones
Hyperthyroidism	Thyroid overworks to produce thyroid hormone due to thyroid hormone resistance by the liver	D(i-3)
Hypothyroidism	Weak thyroid produces less thyroid hormone	D(i-3)
High total cholesterol	Inadequate conversion of cholesterol into steroid hormones by the adrenal gland and sex gland	D(iii)
High LDL cholesterol	Increasing non synthesis of cholesterol from squalene stemming from a weak liver. Squalene is secreted to LDL cholesterol. Hence, a backlog of squalene results in increasing LDL cholesterol	D(iii)
Low HDL cholesterol	Low vitamin D and E due to bile sluggishness	D(iii) – cholesterol D(iv) – bile
Artery plague (atherosclerosis)/ heart disease	Excess backlog of cholesterol over time sticking to artery wall	D(iii)
High blood pressure	Cholesterol plague builds up along artery walls, it slowly blocks the blood flow in the arteries	D(iii)
Kidney problems	Increasing blood pressure together with higher fat & sugar in the blood put a strain on the kidneys	D(iii)
Bad bacteria and toxin build up, imbalance hormones & neurotransmitters	Impaired detoxification	D(iv) – bile D(v) – impaired detoxification
Inflammation and liver insulin resistance (i.e. **high fasting glucose**) leading to diabetes	Free radicals damaging the overworked liver and pancreas	D(i-1) – insulin resistance D(i-2) – diabetes
Liver disease and non-alcoholic fatty liver disease (steatohepatitis)	Accumulation of liver fats arising from bile sluggishness and lower metabolism of fats	D(iv)
Autoimmune diseases	Leaky gut	C(ii)6
Cancer	Low glutathione (due to low glutamine) and low vitamin E and other antioxidants unable to prevent free radical attacks to cell (leading to cell damages) and along with an amplified 5 alpha reductase condition (proliferation of cell). Hence, damaged cell multiplies (cancer)	C(ii-1) – glutathione & glutamine D(iv) – vitamin E A(ii) – 5 alpha reductase

(Left side label: Not so noticeable symptoms)

Figure A(v)1: MetS symptoms and root causes

Note 1:
According to the American Heart Association, to diagnose metabolic syndrome, the presence of three or more of these components are detected:

Components	Measurement
Central obesity	Men – greater than 40 inches (measured by waist circumference)
High triglycerides	Greater than or equal to 150 milligrams per deciliter of blood (mg/dL)
Low HDL cholesterol	Men – less than 40 mg/dL
High blood pressure	Greater than or equal to 130/85 millimetres of mercury (mmHg)
High fasting glucose	Greater than or equal to 100 mg/dL

Figure A(v)2: Diagnostic criteria of MetS according to the American Heart Association - when 3 or more of the above components are detected (which is in line with items highlighted in orange in Figure A(v)1 above). However, according to the author's opinion, these criteria do not capture the full symptoms of MetS

Note 2:
However, manifestation of symptoms differ between people due to differences in nutrition and stress coping styles.

(vi) Borderline Personality Disorder (BPD) or Borderline Depression case study

Variables	Example	Body mechanism	Reference section
Energy (diet) intake	Low glucose, adequate fat, adequate protein, low vitamins, low minerals, low antioxidant food	Adequate protein: less predisposition to endocrine/metabolic issues	C(ii-1) – metabolism D(i) – metabolic issues
		Low glucose: less predisposition to endocrine/metabolic issues, but has trembling/anxiety	C(ii-4) – anxiety D(i)-metabolic issues
		Adequate fat: less predisposition to endocrine/metabolic issues	C(ii-3) – fats D(i) – metabolic issues
		Low vitamins/minerals/antioxidant with *gene problems* (**MTHFR**/MTRR/COMT/MAO-A): *predisposition to methylation issues*	C(i) – methylation
Context & timing of the stress which determine energy redirection & amplification	Low emotional stress [Sadness, anxiety (low serotonin and GABA respectively)] over a relationship breakup	Trigger of energy redirection due to anxiety, hence, predisposition to endocrine/metabolic issue via: • *Cortisol steal*: suppressing sex hormones production in favour of cortisol production • *Conservation of energy*: through slow down digestion of fats • *Catabolisation of protein*: to supply immediate energy for reflex action, depleting our body's protein	A(ii) D(ii) D(iv) C(ii-1)
		Trigger of energy amplification due to anxiety, measured by an *increase in 5 alpha reductase*. *Androgenic* with amplification on both physical and mental traits	A(ii)
Coping style to prevent over exertion	Nutritional intake does not predispose to metabolic issue	No over exertion on physical traits due to adequate nutritional intake, hence, no endocrine/metabolic problem	
	Negative mental coping [low rumination (high oxytocin/dopamine/glutamate)] overworks the brain Also, low vitamins/minerals/antioxidants predispose to methylation impairment	*Low overexertion* of the brain due to low rumination. Overworked brain has higher vibration attracting free radical attacks. *Methylation gene defect expressions* will cause *antioxidant defence against free radical damage to be low*, leading to *low free radical damage* at the brain by impairing glutamate, dopamine, oxytocin receptors, ERβ while triggering *inflammation, oxidative stress* and brain *insulin resistance. Water/nutrients/oxygen cannot be properly absorbed into brain cells.* Without adequate oxygen, *hydroxylation* and brain *oxygen deprivation problems* occur. Brain weakens resulting in brain chemical imbalance (which *cannot be restored to baseline levels due to methylation and oxygen deprivation problems*) thus leading to amplification from borderline normal levels to high levels for oxytocin, glutamate and dopamine while serotonin and GABA are amplified from borderline normal levels toward low levels (BPD or Borderline depression). Refer item (vii) below for all associated symptoms	B – free radical attack C(i) – methylation A Figure A(iii)2 – free radical damage at brain F,G – neurotransmitters, depression F(i-1)4 – BPD/Borderline depression F(i-2)1 – BPD splitting

Figure A(vi)1: BPD or Borderline depression case study: How nutrition, gene predisposition, and stress coping leads to or prevents BPD or Borderline depression

Note: BPD or Borderline depression shares the same key root cause (highlighted in orange above) and impaired body mechanism (highlighted in purple above) with MetS (figure A(iv)1).

(vii) BPD or Borderline depression symptoms & root causes

Symptoms	Root cause	Reference section
Fear of rejection/ abandonment	Very high oxytocin based on bond weakness and low GABA	F(ii) – oxytocin bond, GABA
Jealousy, feeling betrayed/victimised	High to very high level of oxytocin based on distorted perception/memory (arising from a higher to much higher glutamate level) of bond weakness	F(ii) – oxytocin bond, glutamate
Fear or anxiety to being harmed by others	Very low GABA, very high oxytocin based on distorted perception/memory (arising from a higher to much higher glutamate level) of bond weakness	F(ii) – oxytocin bond, GABA, glutamate
Splitting and emotion instability towards others	Variability of oxytocin from normal to very high levels based on distorted perception/memory (arising from a higher to much higher glutamate level) of others' good and bad traits	F(ii) – oxytocin other's traits, glutamate
Aggression/hostility towards others	High to very high level of oxytocin based on distorted perception/memory (arising from a higher to much higher glutamate level) of others' bad traits	F(ii) – oxytocin other's traits, glutamate
Blaming or projection	Very high oxytocin based on distorted perception/memory (arising from a higher to much higher glutamate level) of others' bad traits	F(ii) – oxytocin other's traits, glutamate
Aggression towards self	High to very high level of oxytocin based on distorted perception/memory (arising from a higher to much higher glutamate level) of self's bad traits	F(ii) – oxytocin self's traits, glutamate
Shame, guilt, unworthiness, anger	Variability of oxytocin from high to very high levels based on self's bad traits	F(ii) – oxytocin self's traits
Aggrandization or egotistical	Variability of oxytocin from high to very high levels based on self's good traits	F(ii) – oxytocin self's traits
Unstable identity, boredom & feeling empty or lost	Damaged to prefrontal cortex in correlation with dopamine (Link 20)	F(ii) – dopamine
Impulsivity	High to higher dopamine	F(ii) – dopamine
Changing goals	Easily change goals when frustrated (low to very low serotonin & high to higher dopamine)	F(ii) – dopamine, serotonin
Feeling loss of gratification and frustration	High to higher dopamine levels where reward is not reinforced and low to very low serotonin	F(ii) – dopamine, serotonin
Anxiety, irritability & depression	Low GABA and low to very low serotonin	F(ii) – serotonin, GABA
Feeling overwhelmed	Increases in stress chemical levels such as dopamine, adrenaline and noradrenaline arising from a decrease in COMT activity. Correlates with high to higher dopamine	F(i-2) F(ii) – dopamine
Mouth muscle twitch	Low GABA (muscle spasm), refer (Link 21)	F(ii) – GABA
Paranoia and Dysphoria	Very low GABA (Link 22)	F(ii) – GABA
Dissociation	Very low GABA and wrong perception & memory (much higher glutamate) (Link 23)	F(ii) – GABA, glutamate
Cognition/perception/memory problems	Neurotoxin arising from higher to much higher glutamate	F(ii) – glutamate
Psychosis	Very high glutamate or dopamine	F(ii) – glutamate, dopamine

Figure A(vii)1: Borderline Personality Disorder (BPD) or Borderline Depression symptoms (with reference from Note 2 below) and root causes

Note 1: Based on the above root causes, it can be seen that the BPD symptoms arise due to fluctuating neurotransmitters between normal levels and amplified very high levels for oxytocin, dopamine, glutamate while serotonin and GABA are amplified toward very low levels.

However, manifestation of symptoms differ between people due to differences in nutrition and stress coping styles.

Note 2:

BPD symptoms according to literature

- *Frantic efforts to avoid abandonment*, whether the abandonment is real or imagined. The most distinguishing symptoms of BPD are marked *sensitivity to rejection or criticism, and intense fear of possible abandonment* [(Link 24) and (Link 25)].

- *A pattern of unstable and intense interpersonal relationships characterized by alternating between extremes of idealization and devaluation (splitting)*. People with BPD can be very sensitive to the way others treat them, by feeling intense joy and gratitude at perceived expressions of kindness, and intense sadness or anger at perceived criticism or hurtfulness. Their feelings about others often shift from admiration or love to anger or dislike after a disappointment, a threat of losing someone, or a perceived loss of esteem in the eyes of someone they value. *While strongly desiring intimacy, people with BPD tend toward insecure, avoidant or ambivalent, or fearfully preoccupied attachment patterns in relationships and they often view the world as dangerous and malevolent* (Link 26).

- *Identity disturbance and chronic feelings of emptiness*, such as a significant and persistent unstable self-image or sense of self. Tend to have trouble seeing a clear picture of their identity. In particular, they tend to have difficulty knowing what they value, believe, prefer, and enjoy. They are often unsure about their long-term goals for relationships and jobs. This difficulty with knowing who they are and what they value can cause people with BPD to experience *feeling "empty" and "lost"*.

- *Impulsivity* in at least two areas that are potentially self-damaging (e.g. spending, sex, substance abuse, reckless driving, binge eating, *running away, leaving jobs, leaving relationships*) to relieve emotional pain.

- *Emotional instability* due to significant reactivity of mood (e.g. *intense episodic dysphoria, irritability, or anxiety usually lasting a few hours and only rarely more than a few days*). Intense or uncontrollable emotional reactions that often seem disproportionate to the situation. People with BPD feel emotions more easily, more deeply, and longer than others do. In addition, *emotions may repeatedly resurge and persist a long time*. While people with BPD feel joy intensely, they are especially *prone to dysphoria, depression, and/or feelings of mental and emotional distress*.
    - Zanarini et al. recognized four categories of dysphoria that are typical of this condition: extreme emotions, destructiveness or self-destructiveness, feeling fragmented or lacking identity, and feelings of victimization.
    - Within these categories, a BPD diagnosis is strongly associated with a combination of three specific states: *feeling betrayed, "feeling like hurting myself", and feeling out of control*.

- *Inappropriate, intense anger* or difficulty controlling anger (e.g. frequent displays of temper, constant anger, recurrent physical fights). People with BPD are *prone to feeling angry at members of their family* and are alienated from them.

- *Transient, stress-related paranoid thoughts* (e.g. generally used to refer to intense beliefs of mistrust or the malicious intentions of others, for example, *feel people are out to use/cheat/abuse/oppress/harm*) or severe dissociative symptoms (feeling "out of it," or *not being able to remember what they said or did. This mostly happens in times of severe stress*) (Link 27).

- *Recurrent suicidal or self-damaging behaviour/gestures, or threats, or self-mutilating behaviour*.

With reference from: (Link 28), (Link 29) and Diagnostic & Statistical Manual of Mental Disorders (DSM) version 5.

Note 3:

<u>Borderline Personality Disorder (BPD) vs. Major Depression</u>

Having to endure the stress of BPD symptoms, Borderliners can fall into depression. However, their quality of depression defers from Major Depression (MDD).

(Link 30) lists the qualitative difference between the symptoms of MDD and those of depressed people with BPD. The quality of their depression is characterized by the following:

- *A "mad-bad" depression closely tied to anger and hostile behaviour*.

- Mood symptoms that are very sensitive to interpersonal situations in which the patient *feels abandoned, lonely, or empty in the absence [or in the presence for that matter] of a longed-for important other*.

- Depressed moods can come on quickly and disappear quickly *[the opposite of true MDD]* depending on the reactions of an attachment figure.

- The depression is at times more closely related to chronic self-criticism and a feeling of intrinsic "badness" than in MDD without BPD.

- It is associated with chronic self-destructive behaviour *[including self-injurious behaviour like cutting]*.

- It is associated with a loss of gratification and frustration.

- *Recovery from BPD facilitates recovery from MDD when it is co-occurring, rather than the other way around*.

- *The depression often comes from exhaustion and demoralization from repeated unsuccessful battles with chronic and overwhelming anxiety. [BPD is often accompanied by panic disorder]*.

- Borderliners often exhibit *impulsive aggression* (a hair trigger leading to rage). *[Patients with true major depression, especially of the melancholic variety, tend not to show this characteristic at all. They are usually extremely passive because they do not have the energy to strike out]*.

- Normally BPD and MDD co-occur together but often times, the *BPD diagnosis is missed out*.

- Borderline Personality Disorder can be inherited. *Heritability is estimated at 40%*.

Author's opinion:
BPD diagnosis is often misdiagnosed due to the interchangeability of the mood disorders along the mania-depression spectrum, refer A(iii)8.

(viii) Dysthymia case study

Variables	Example	Body mechanism	Reference section
Energy (diet) intake	Low glucose, adequate fat, adequate protein, low vitamins, low minerals, low antioxidant food	Adequate protein: less predisposition to endocrine/metabolic issues	C(ii-1) – metabolism D(i) – metabolic issues
		Low glucose: less predisposition to endocrine/metabolic issues, but has trembling/anxiety	C(ii-4) – anxiety D(i) – metabolic issues
		Adequate fat: less predisposition to endocrine/metabolic issues	C(ii-3) – fats D(i) – metabolic issues
		Low vitamins/minerals/antioxidant with *gene problems* (**MTHFR**/MTRR/COMT/MAO-A): *predisposition to methylation issues*	C(i) – methylation
Context & timing of the stress which determine energy redirection & amplification	**Moderate emotional stress** [Sadness, feeling slightly unworthy, anxious & hopeless (low serotonin/ oxytocin/ GABA/ dopamine respectively)] on a daily basis	Trigger of energy redirection due to anxiety, hence, predisposition to endocrine/metabolic issue via: • *Cortisol steal*: suppressing sex hormones production in favour of cortisol production • *Conservation of energy:* through slow down digestion of fats • *Catabolisation of protein:* to supply immediate energy for reflex action, depleting our body's protein	A(ii) D(ii) D(iv) C(ii-1)
		Trigger of energy amplification due to anxiety, measured by an *increase in 5 alpha reductase*. *Androgenic* with amplification on both physical and mental traits	A(ii)
Coping style to prevent over exertion	Nutritional intake does not predispose to metabolic issue	No over exertion on physical traits due to adequate nutritional intake, hence, no endocrine/metabolic problem	
	Negative mental coping [**moderate rumination** (moderately higher oxytocin, dopamine, glutamate)] overworks brain Also, low vitamins/minerals/ antioxidants predispose to methylation impairment	*Moderate overexertion* of the brain due to moderate rumination. Overworked brain has higher vibration attracting free radical attacks. *Methylation gene defect expressions* will cause *antioxidant defence against free radical damage to be low,* leading to *moderate free radical damage* at the brain by impairing glutamate, dopamine, oxytocin receptors, ERβ while triggering *inflammation, oxidative stress* and brain *insulin resistance. Water/nutrients/oxygen cannot be properly absorbed into brain cells.* Without adequate oxygen, *hydroxylation* and brain *oxygen deprivation problems* occur. Brain weakens resulting in brain chemical imbalance (which *cannot be restored to baseline levels due to methylation and oxygen deprivation problems*) thus leading to low levels of dopamine, oxytocin, GABA, glutamate and serotonin (Dysthymia). Refer item (ix) below for all associated symptoms	B – free radical attack C(i) – methylation A Figure A(iii)3 – free radical damage at brain F,G – neurotransmitters, depression F(i-2)4 – dysthymia

Figure A(viii)1: Dysthymia case study: How nutrition, gene predisposition, and stress coping leads to or prevents Dysthymia

Note: Dysthymia shares the same key root cause (highlighted in orange above) and impaired body mechanism (highlighted in purple above) with MetS (figure A(iv)1).

(ix) *Dysthymia symptoms & root causes*

Symptoms	Root cause	Reference section
Fatigue or loss of energy	Total brain energy level is severely inhibiting	F(iii-a)
A depressed & irritable mood almost every day for most of the day	Low GABA and low serotonin	F(ii) – serotonin, GABA
Having a poor appetite	Low serotonin	F(ii) – serotonin
Sleep disturbance	Low serotonin	F(ii) – serotonin F(i-1) – melatonin
Low self esteem	Low oxytocin where there is low focus on self's good traits	F(ii) – oxytocin self's traits
Poor concentration or difficulty making decisions	Low glutamate	F(ii) – glutamate
Feelings of hopelessness	Low dopamine	F(ii) – dopamine

Figure A(ix)1: Dysthymia symptoms [according to Diagnostic and Statistical Manual of Mental Disorders (DSM) version 5] and root causes

Note 1: Based on the above root causes, it can be seen that the Dysthymia symptoms arise due to low levels for oxytocin, dopamine, glutamate, GABA and serotonin.

Note 2: Dysthymia is a chronic but less severe form of Major depression (also known as persistent depressive disorder or PDD). Dysthymia can lasts for years.

However, manifestation of symptoms differ between people due to differences in nutrition and stress coping styles.

(x) Bipolar case study

Variables	Example	Body mechanism	Reference section
Energy (diet) intake	Low glucose, adequate fat, excessive protein, low vitamins, low minerals, low antioxidant food	Excessive protein: less predisposition to endocrine/metabolic issues but elevated tryptophan (precursor to serotonin) and tyrosine (precursor to dopamine), predisposition to high arousal, affect and energy level	C(ii-1) – metabolism D(i) – metabolic issues
		Low glucose: less predisposition to endocrine/metabolic issues, but has trembling/anxiety	C(ii-4) – anxiety D(i) – metabolic issues
		Adequate fat: less predisposition to endocrine/metabolic issues	C(ii-3) – fats D(i) – metabolic issues
		Low vitamins/minerals/antioxidant with *gene problems* (**MTHFR**/MTRR/COMT/MAO-A): *predisposition to methylation issues*	C(i) – methylation
Context & timing of the stress which determine energy redirection & amplification	**Moderate emotional stress** [Frustrated, anxious (low serotonin & GABA respectively) and angry, feeling unappreciated (high oxytocin & dopamine respectively)] over a relationship breakup	Trigger of energy redirection due to anxiety, hence, predisposition to endocrine/metabolic issue via: • *Cortisol steal*: suppressing sex hormones production in favour of cortisol production • *Conservation of energy*: through slow down digestion of fats • *Catabolisation of protein*: to supply immediate energy for reflex action, depleting our body's protein	A(ii) D(ii) D(iv) C(ii-1)
		Trigger of energy amplification due to anxiety, measured by an *increase in 5 alpha reductase*. *Androgenic* with amplification on both physical and mental traits	A(ii)
Coping style to prevent over exertion	Nutritional intake does not predispose to metabolic issue	No over exertion on physical traits due to adequate nutritional intake, hence, no endocrine/metabolic problem	
	Negative mental coping [**moderate rumination** (moderately higher oxytocin/dopamine/glutamate)] overworks the brain Also, low vitamins/minerals/antioxidants predispose to methylation impairment	Initially, *low overexertion* of the brain due to low rumination. Overworked brain has higher vibration attracting free radical attacks. *Methylation gene defect expressions* will cause *antioxidant defence against free radical damage to be low*, leading to *low free radical damage* at the brain by impairing glutamate, dopamine, oxytocin receptors, ERβ while triggering *inflammation, oxidative stress* and brain *insulin resistance*. *Water/nutrients/oxygen cannot be properly absorbed into brain cells*. Without adequate oxygen, *hydroxylation* and brain *oxygen deprivation problems* occur. Brain weakens resulting in brain chemical imbalance (which *cannot be restored to baseline levels due to methylation and oxygen deprivation problems*) thus leading to amplification from borderline levels to high levels for oxytocin, glutamate and dopamine while serotonin and GABA are amplified from borderline levels toward very low levels (BPD or Borderline depression).	B – free radical attack C(i) – methylation A Figure A(iii)2 – free radical damage at brain F,G – neurotransmitters, depression
	Moderately excessive protein intake level elevates serotonin and dopamine	However, due to increasing moderate emotional stress, moderate rumination & moderately excessive protein intake level, the borderline depression is now transformed into Bipolar II where both serotonin and dopamine are further elevated. This leads to a very high level for dopamine, high levels for oxytocin, glutamate, baseline	F(iii-b) – Bipolar F(i-2)2 – Bipolar hypomania-mania

		normal level for serotonin and low level for GABA (Bipolar hypomania phase)	
		However, an overly excited brain will attract free radical attacks, *resulting in high free radical damages and high overexertion of the brain* that can lead to all neurotransmitters being depressed (Bipolar moderate depression phase)	F(i-2)3 – Bipolar moderate-major depression

A Figure A(iii)4 – free radical damage at brain |
| | | Refer item (xi) below for all associated symptoms | |

Figure A(x)1: Bipolar II case study: How nutrition, gene predisposition, and stress coping leads to or prevents Bipolar

Note: Bipolar shares the same key root cause (highlighted in orange above) and impaired body mechanism (highlighted in purple above) with MetS (figure A(iv)1).

(xi) *Bipolar symptoms & root causes*

Symptoms	Root cause	Reference section
Grandiosity/an inflated sense of self	High oxytocin based on self's good traits	F(ii) – Oxytocin self's traits
Little need for sleep	Total brain energy is excitatory (high energy level) and serotonin is at baseline normal level. Hence, a lot of energy without need for sleep	F(iii-b) – Bipolar
F(ii) – Serotonin
Increased rate of speech (talking fast, loudly, rapidly)	Total brain energy is excitatory (high energy level) and high glutamate	F(iii-b) – Bipolar
F(ii) – Glutamate
Flight of ideas/ racing thoughts	Total brain energy is excitatory (high energy level) and high glutamate	F(iii-b) – Bipolar
F(ii) – Glutamate
Getting easily distracted	Very high dopamine, baseline normal level for serotonin	F(ii) – Dopamine
F(ii) – Serotonin
An increased interest in goals and activities/ engaging in multiple tasks at one time (more than can be realistically accomplished in a day)	Very high dopamine	F(ii) – Dopamine
Psychomotor agitation (i.e. pacing around the room, tapping toes, rapid talking), where it normally occurs with anxiety or mania	Low GABA, very high dopamine	F(ii) – GABA
F(ii) – Dopamine
Increased pursuit of activities with a high risk of danger	Very high dopamine	F(ii) – Dopamine

Figure A(xi)1: Bipolar hypomania-mania symptoms [according to Diagnostic and Statistical Manual of Mental Disorders (DSM) version 5] and root causes. The symptoms for hypomania are less in severity compared to mania

Note: Based on the above root causes, it can be seen that the Bipolar hypomania-mania symptoms arise due to very high level for dopamine, high levels for oxytocin & glutamate, baseline normal level for serotonin and low level for GABA.

Symptoms	Root cause	Reference section
Moderate – major depression where symptoms are similar to A(xiii)1	Free radical attacks on an overexcited brain	F(iii-b) – Bipolar

Figure A(xi)2: Bipolar moderate-major depression symptoms and root causes. The symptoms for moderate depression are less in severity compared to major depression

Note: Based on the above root causes, it can be seen that the Bipolar moderate-major depression symptoms arise due to low levels for oxytocin, dopamine, glutamate, GABA and moderate to very low level for serotonin.

However, manifestation of bipolar symptoms differ between people due to differences in nutrition and stress coping styles.

(xii) Major depression with anxiety case study

Variables	Example	Body mechanism	Reference section
Energy (diet) intake	Low glucose, adequate fat, adequate protein, low vitamins, low minerals, low antioxidant food	Adequate protein: less predisposition to endocrine/metabolic issues	C(ii-1) – metabolism D(i) – metabolic issues
		Low glucose: less predisposition to endocrine/metabolic issues, but has trembling/anxiety	C(ii-4) – anxiety D(i) – metabolic issues
		Adequate fat: less predisposition to endocrine/metabolic issues	C(ii-3) – fats D(i) – metabolic issues
		Low vitamins/minerals/antioxidant with *gene problems* (**MTHFR**/MTRR/COMT/MAO-A): *predisposition to methylation issues*	C(i) – methylation
Context & timing of the stress which determine energy redirection & amplification	Extreme emotional stress [Grief, feeling unworthy, anxious, hopeless (very low serotonin & low oxytocin, GABA and dopamine respectively)] over a divorce	Trigger of energy redirection due to anxiety, hence, predisposition to endocrine/metabolic issue via: • *Cortisol steal*: suppressing sex hormones production in favour of cortisol production • *Conservation of energy*: through slow down digestion of fats • *Catabolisation of protein*: to supply immediate energy for reflex action, depleting our body's protein	A(ii) D(ii) D(iv) C(ii-1)
		Trigger of energy amplification due to anxiety, measured by an *increase in 5 alpha reductase*. *Androgenic* with amplification on both physical and mental traits	A(ii)
Coping style to prevent over exertion	Nutritional intake does not predispose to metabolic issue	No over exertion on physical traits due to adequate nutritional intake, hence, no endocrine/metabolic problem	
	Negative mental coping [extreme rumination (very high oxytocin, dopamine, glutamate)] overworks brain. Also, low vitamins/minerals/antioxidants predispose to methylation impairment	*Extreme overexertion* of the brain due to extreme rumination. Overworked brain has higher vibration attracting free radical attacks. *Methylation gene defect expressions* will cause *antioxidant defence against free radical damage to be low*, leading to *extreme free radical damage* at the brain by impairing glutamate, dopamine, oxytocin receptors, ERβ while triggering *inflammation, oxidative stress* and brain *insulin resistance. Water/nutrients/oxygen cannot be properly absorbed into brain cells.* Without adequate oxygen, *hydroxylation* and brain *oxygen deprivation problems* occur. Brain weakens resulting in brain chemical imbalance (which *cannot be restored to baseline levels due to methylation and oxygen deprivation problems*) thus leading to low levels of dopamine, oxytocin, GABA, glutamate and very low level for serotonin (Major depression with anxiety). Refer item (xiii) below for all associated symptoms	B – free radical attack C(i) – methylation A Figure A(iii)5 – free radical damage at brain F,G – neurotransmitters, depression F(i-1)3 – major depression with anxiety

Figure A(xii)1: Major depression with anxiety case study: How nutrition, gene predisposition, and stress coping leads to or prevents Major depression with anxiety

Note: Major depression with anxiety shares the same key root cause (highlighted in orange above) and impaired body mechanism (highlighted in purple above) with MetS (figure A(iv)1).

(xiii) *Major depression with anxiety symptoms & root causes*

Symptoms	Root cause	Reference section
Fatigue or loss of energy	Total brain energy level is severely inhibiting	F(iii-a)
Anxiety, irritability & depression	Low GABA and low to very low serotonin	F(ii) – serotonin, GABA
Significant weight change or appetite disturbance	Very low serotonin	F(ii) – serotonin
Sleep disturbance	Very low serotonin	F(ii) – serotonin F(i-1) – melatonin
Diminished interest or loss of pleasure in almost all activities (anhedonia)	Low dopamine	F(ii) – dopamine
Psychomotor agitation (i.e. pacing around the room, tapping toes, rapid talking), where it normally occurs with anxiety or mania	Low GABA	F(ii) – GABA
Diminished ability to think or concentrate; indecisiveness	Low glutamate	F(ii) – glutamate
Recurrent thoughts of death/ recurrent suicidal ideation (Aggression towards self)	Total brain energy level is severely inhibiting, low level of oxytocin based on distorted perception/memory (arising from a low glutamate level) of self's good traits	F(iii-a) F(ii) – oxytocin self's traits, glutamate
Lack of worthiness, loss of confidence	Low oxytocin where there is low focus on self's good traits	F(ii) – oxytocin self's traits

Figure A(xiii)1: Major depression with anxiety symptoms [according to Diagnostic and Statistical Manual of Mental Disorders (DSM) version 5] and root causes

Note 1: Based on the above root causes, it can be seen that the Major depression with anxiety symptoms arise due to low levels for oxytocin, dopamine, glutamate, GABA and very low level for serotonin.

However, manifestation of symptoms differ between people due to differences in nutrition and stress coping styles.

Radical theory on MetS & Depression

(xiv) <u>MetS with Borderline Personality Disorder (BPD) or Borderline Depression case study</u>

Variables	Example	Body mechanism	Reference section
Energy (diet) intake	Diet of high simple glucose, high bad fat, low protein, low vitamins, low minerals and low antioxidant	Low protein: predisposition to endocrine/metabolic issues	C(ii-1) – metabolism D(i) – metabolic issues
		High simple glucose: predisposition to endocrine/metabolic issues, high free radicals	C(ii-2) – excess glucose D(i) – metabolic issues B – free radical
		Excess bad fat: predisposition to endocrine/metabolic issues	C(ii-3) – fats D(i) – metabolic issues
		Low vitamins/minerals/antioxidant with *gene problems* (MTHFR/MTRR/COMT/MAO-A): *predisposition to methylation issues*	C(i) – methylation
Context & timing of the stress which determine energy redirection & amplification	Extreme anxiety (low GABA) to achieve work deadlines overworks the liver Low emotional stress [Sadness, anxiety (low serotonin and GABA respectively)] over a relationship breakup	Trigger of energy redirection due to anxiety, hence, predisposition to endocrine/metabolic issue via: • *Cortisol steal*: suppressing sex hormones production in favour of cortisol production • *Conservation of energy:* through slow down digestion of fats • *Catabolisation of protein:* to supply immediate energy for reflex action, depleting our body's protein Trigger of energy amplification due to anxiety, measured by an *increase in 5 alpha reductase*. *Androgenic* with amplification on both physical and mental traits	A(ii) D(ii) D(iv) C(ii-1) A(ii)
Coping style to prevent over exertion	Extreme bad diet: Low protein, bad fats and high glucose intake unable to support liver functions in stress handling Also, low vitamins/minerals/antioxidants predispose to methylation impairment Negative mental coping [low rumination (high oxytocin/ dopamine/ glutamate)] overworks the brain Also, low vitamins/minerals/antioxidants	*Extreme overexertion* of the liver to support extreme anxious stress handling. Overworked liver has higher vibration attracting free radical attacks. *Methylation gene defect expression* will cause *antioxidant defence against free radical damages to be low*, leading to *extreme free radical damage* at the liver (ERα) and triggering *inflammation, oxidative stress* & liver *insulin resistance*. Thus, *water/nutrients/oxygen cannot be properly absorbed into liver cells*, impairing liver's *hydroxylation* process. Liver weakens resulting in a hormonal imbalance (which *cannot be restored to baseline levels due to methylation and oxygen deprivation problems*) thus leading to MetS, infertility. Refer item (v) above for all associated symptoms *Low overexertion* of the brain due to low rumination. Overworked brain has higher vibration attracting free radical attacks. *Methylation gene defect expressions* will cause *antioxidant defence against free radical damage to be low*, leading to *low free radical damage* at the brain by impairing glutamate, dopamine, oxytocin receptors, ERβ while triggering *inflammation, oxidative stress* and brain *insulin resistance. Water/nutrients/oxygen cannot be properly absorbed into brain cells.* Without adequate oxygen, *hydroxylation* and brain *oxygen deprivation problems* occur. Brain weakens resulting in brain chemical	B – free radical attack C(i) – methylation A Figure A(iii)1 – free radical damage at liver D – impact of free radical damage on neuroendocrine B – free radical attack C(i) – methylation A Figure A(iii)2 – free radical damage at brain F,G – neurotransmitters, depression

| | predispose to methylation impairment | imbalance (which *cannot be restored to baseline levels due to methylation and oxygen deprivation problems*) thus leading to amplification from borderline normal levels to high levels for oxytocin, glutamate and dopamine while serotonin and GABA are amplified from borderline normal levels toward low levels (BPD or Borderline depression). Refer item (vii) above for all associated symptoms | F(i-1)4 – BPD/Borderline depression

F(i-2)1 – BPD splitting |

Figure A(xiv)1: MetS with BPD or Borderline depression case study: How nutrition, gene predisposition, and stress coping leads to or prevents MetS with BPD or Borderline depression

(xv) MetS with Dysthymia case study

Variables	Example	Body mechanism	Reference section
Energy (diet) intake	Diet of high simple glucose, high bad fat, low protein, low vitamins, low minerals and low antioxidant	Low protein: predisposition to endocrine/metabolic issues	C(ii-1) – metabolism D(i) – metabolic issues
		High simple glucose: predisposition to endocrine/metabolic issues, high free radicals	C(ii-2) – excess glucose D(i) – metabolic issues B – free radical
		Excess bad fat: predisposition to endocrine/metabolic issues	C(ii-3) – fats D(i) – metabolic issues
		Low vitamins/minerals/antioxidant with *gene problems* (MTHFR/MTRR/COMT/MAO-A): *predisposition to methylation issues*	C(i) – methylation
Context & timing of the stress which determine energy redirection & amplification	**Extreme anxiety** (low GABA) to achieve work deadlines overworks the liver **Moderate emotional stress** [Sadness, feeling slightly unworthy, anxious & hopeless (low serotonin/ oxytocin/ GABA/ dopamine respectively)] on a daily basis	Trigger of energy redirection due to anxiety, hence, predisposition to endocrine/metabolic issue via: • *Cortisol steal:* suppressing sex hormones production in favour of cortisol production • *Conservation of energy:* through slow down digestion of fats • *Catabolisation of protein:* to supply immediate energy for reflex action, depleting our body's protein Trigger of energy amplification due to anxiety, measured by an *increase in 5 alpha reductase*. *Androgenic* with amplification on both physical and mental traits	A(ii) D(ii) D(iv) C(ii-1) A(ii)
Coping style to prevent over exertion	**Extreme bad diet**: Low protein, bad fats and high glucose intake unable to support liver functions in stress handling Also, low vitamins/minerals/ antioxidants predispose to methylation impairment	*Extreme overexertion* of the liver to support extreme anxious stress handling. Overworked liver has higher vibration attracting free radical attacks. *Methylation gene defect expression* will cause *antioxidant defence against free radical damages to be low*, leading to *extreme free radical damage* at the liver (ERα) and triggering *inflammation, oxidative stress* & liver *insulin resistance*. Thus, *water/nutrients/oxygen cannot be properly absorbed into liver cells*, impairing liver's *hydroxylation* process. Liver weakens resulting in a hormonal imbalance (which *cannot be restored to baseline levels due to methylation and oxygen deprivation problems*) thus leading to MetS, infertility. Refer item (v) above for all associated symptoms	B – free radical attack C(i) – methylation A Figure A(iii)1 – free radical damage at liver D – impact of free radical damage on neuroendocrine
	Negative mental coping [**moderate rumination** (moderately higher oxytocin, dopamine, glutamate)] overworks brain	*Moderate overexertion* of the brain due to moderate rumination. Overworked brain has higher vibration attracting free radical attacks. *Methylation gene defect expressions* will cause *antioxidant defence against free radical damage to be low*, leading to *moderate free radical damage* at the brain by impairing glutamate, dopamine, oxytocin receptors, ERβ while triggering *inflammation, oxidative stress* and brain *insulin resistance*. *Water/nutrients/oxygen cannot be properly absorbed into brain cells*. Without adequate	B – free radical attack C(i) – methylation A Figure A(iii)3 – free radical damage at brain F,G – neurotransmitters, depression

| | Also, low vitamins/minerals/ antioxidants predispose to methylation impairment | oxygen, *hydroxylation* and brain *oxygen deprivation problems* occur. Brain weakens resulting in brain chemical imbalance (which *cannot be restored to baseline levels due to methylation and oxygen deprivation problems*) thus leading to low levels of dopamine, oxytocin, GABA, glutamate and serotonin (Dysthymia). Refer item (ix) above for all associated symptoms | F(i-2)4 – dysthymia |

Figure A(xv)1: MetS with Dysthymia case study: How nutrition, gene predisposition, and stress coping leads to or prevents MetS with Dysthymia

(xvi) MetS with Bipolar case study

Variables	Example	Body mechanism	Reference section
Energy (diet) intake	Diet of high simple glucose, high bad fat, excess protein, low vitamins, low minerals and low antioxidant	Excessive protein: less predisposition to endocrine/metabolic issues but elevated tryptophan (precursor to serotonin) and tyrosine (precursor to dopamine), predisposition to high arousal, affect and energy level	C(ii-1) – metabolism D(i) – metabolic issues
		High simple glucose: predisposition to endocrine/ metabolic issues, high free radicals	C(ii-2) – excess glucose D(i) – metabolic issues B – free radical
		Excess bad fat: predisposition to endocrine/metabolic issues	C(ii-3) – fats D(i) – metabolic issues
		Low vitamins/minerals/antioxidant with *gene problems* (*MTHFR*/MTRR/COMT/MAO-A): *predisposition to methylation issues*	C(i) – methylation
Context & timing of the stress which determine energy redirection & amplification	**Extreme anxiety** (low GABA) to achieve work deadlines overworks the liver **Moderate emotional stress** [Frustrated, anxious (low serotonin & GABA respectively) and angry, feeling unappreciated (high oxytocin & dopamine respectively)] over a relationship breakup	Trigger of energy redirection due to anxiety, hence, predisposition to endocrine/metabolic issue via: • *Cortisol steal*: suppressing sex hormones production in favour of cortisol production • *Conservation of energy:* through slow down digestion of fats • *Catabolisation of protein:* to supply immediate energy for reflex action, depleting our body's protein Trigger of energy amplification due to anxiety, measured by an *increase in 5 alpha reductase. Androgenic* with amplification on both physical and mental traits	A(ii) D(ii) D(iv) C(ii-1) A(ii)
Coping style to prevent over exertion	**Extreme bad diet**: Bad fats and high glucose intake unable to support liver functions in stress handling Also, low vitamins /minerals/ antioxidants predispose to methylation impairment Negative mental coping [**moderate rumination**	*Extreme overexertion* of the liver to support extreme anxious stress handling. Overworked liver has higher vibration attracting free radical attacks. *Methylation gene defect expression* will cause *antioxidant defence against free radical damages to be low*, leading to *extreme free radical damage* at the liver (ERα) and triggering *inflammation, oxidative stress* & liver *insulin resistance*. Thus, *water/nutrients/oxygen cannot be properly absorbed into liver cells*, impairing liver's *hydroxylation* process. Liver weakens resulting in a hormonal imbalance (which *cannot be restored to baseline levels due to methylation and oxygen deprivation problems*) thus leading to MetS, infertility. Refer item (v) above for all associated symptoms Initially, *low overexertion* of the brain due to low rumination. Overworked brain has higher vibration attracting free radical attacks. *Methylation gene defect*	B – free radical attack C(i) – methylation A Figure A(iii)1 – free radical damage at liver D – impact of free radical damage on neuroendocrine B – free radical attack C(i) – methylation

	(moderately higher oxytocin/ dopamine/ glutamate)] overworks the brain

Also, low vitamins/ minerals/ antioxidants predispose to methylation impairment | *expressions* will cause **antioxidant defence against free radical damage to be low**, leading to *low free radical damage* at the brain by impairing glutamate, dopamine, oxytocin receptors, ERβ while triggering **inflammation, oxidative stress** and brain **insulin resistance. Water/nutrients/oxygen cannot be properly absorbed into brain cells.** Without adequate oxygen, *hydroxylation* and brain *oxygen deprivation problems* occur. Brain weakens resulting in brain chemical imbalance (which *cannot be restored to baseline levels due to methylation and oxygen deprivation problems*) thus leading to amplification from borderline levels to high levels for oxytocin, glutamate and dopamine while serotonin and GABA are amplified from borderline levels toward low levels (BPD or Borderline depression) | A Figure A(iii)2 – free radical damage at brain

F,G – neurotransmitters, depression |
| | **Moderately excessive protein intake level** elevates serotonin and dopamine | However, due to increasing moderate emotional stress, moderate rumination & moderately excessive protein intake level, the borderline depression is now transformed into Bipolar II where both serotonin and dopamine are further elevated. This leads to a very high level for dopamine, high levels for oxytocin, glutamate, baseline normal level for serotonin and low level for GABA (Bipolar hypomania phase) | F(iii-b) – Bipolar

F(i-2)2 – Bipolar hypomania-mania |
| | | However, an overly excited brain will attract free radical attacks, *resulting in high free radical damages and high overexertion of the brain* that can lead to all neurotransmitters being depressed (Bipolar moderate depression phase)

Refer item (xi) above for all associated symptoms | F(i-2)3 – Bipolar moderate-major depression

A Figure A(iii)4 – free radical damage at brain |

Figure A(xvi)1: MetS with Bipolar II case study: How nutrition, gene predisposition, and stress coping leads to or prevents MetS with Bipolar

(xvii) MetS with Major depression & anxiety case study

Variables	Example	Body mechanism	Reference section
Energy (diet) intake	Diet of high simple glucose, high bad fat, low protein, low vitamins, low minerals and low antioxidant	Low protein: predisposition to endocrine/metabolic issues	C(ii-1) – metabolism D(i) – metabolic issues
		High simple glucose: predisposition to endocrine/metabolic issues, high free radicals	C(ii-2) – excess glucose D(i) – metabolic issues B – free radical
		Excess bad fat: predisposition to endocrine/metabolic issues	C(ii-3) – fats D(i) – metabolic issues
		Low vitamins/minerals/antioxidant with *gene problems* (**MTHFR**/MTRR/COMT/MAO-A): *predisposition to methylation issues*	C(i) – methylation
Context & timing of the stress which determine energy redirection & amplification	**Extreme anxiety** (low GABA) to achieve work deadlines overworks the liver **Extreme emotional stress** [Grief, feeling unworthy, anxious, hopeless (very low serotonin & low oxytocin, GABA and dopamine respectively)] over a divorce	Trigger of energy redirection due to anxiety, hence, predisposition to endocrine/metabolic issue via: • *Cortisol steal*: suppressing sex hormones production in favour of cortisol production • *Conservation of energy:* through slow down digestion of fats • *Catabolisation of protein*: to supply immediate energy for reflex action, depleting our body's protein Trigger of energy amplification due to anxiety, measured by an *increase in 5 alpha reductase*. *Androgenic* with amplification on both physical and mental traits	A(ii) D(ii) D(iv) C(ii-1) A(ii)
Coping style to prevent over exertion	**Extreme bad diet**: Low protein, bad fats and high glucose intake unable to support liver functions in stress handling Also, low vitamins/minerals/antioxidants predispose to methylation impairment	*Extreme overexertion* of the liver to support extreme anxious stress handling. Overworked liver has higher vibration attracting free radical attacks. *Methylation gene defect expression* will cause *antioxidant defence against free radical damages to be low*, leading to *extreme free radical damage* at the liver (ERα) and triggering *inflammation, oxidative stress* & liver *insulin resistance*. Thus, *water/nutrients/oxygen cannot be properly absorbed into liver cells*, impairing liver's *hydroxylation* process. Liver weakens resulting in a hormonal imbalance (which *cannot be restored to baseline levels due to methylation and oxygen deprivation problems*) thus leading to MetS, infertility. Refer item (v) above for all associated symptoms	B – free radical attack C(i) – methylation A Figure A(iii)1 – free radical damage at liver D – impact of free radical damage on neuroendocrine
	Negative mental coping [**extreme rumination** [very high oxytocin, dopamine, glutamate] overworks the brain	*Extreme overexertion* of the brain due to extreme rumination. Overworked brain has higher vibration attracting free radical attacks. *Methylation gene defect expressions* will cause *antioxidant defence against free radical damage to be low*, leading to *extreme free radical damage* at the brain by impairing glutamate, dopamine, oxytocin receptors, ERβ while triggering *inflammation, oxidative stress* and brain *insulin resistance. Water/nutrients/oxygen cannot be properly*	B – free radical attack C(i) – methylation A Figure A(iii)5 – free radical damage at brain

| | Also, low vitamins/minerals/ antioxidants predispose to methylation impairment | *absorbed into brain cells.* Without adequate oxygen, *hydroxylation* and brain *oxygen deprivation problems* occur. Brain weakens resulting in brain chemical imbalance (which *cannot be restored to baseline levels due to methylation and oxygen deprivation problems*) thus leading to low levels of dopamine, oxytocin, GABA, glutamate and very low level of serotonin (Major depression with anxiety). Refer item (xiii) above for all associated symptoms | F,G – neurotransmitters, depression F(i-1)3 – major depression with anxiety |

Figure A(xvii)1: MetS with Major depression & anxiety case study: How nutrition, gene predisposition, and stress coping leads to or prevents MetS with Major depression & anxiety

(xviii) Common root causes and impaired body mechanism between MetS and Depression

04 Weakened cells & organs (as per item 03) unable to restore chemical balance (either hormone or brain chemical) to baseline levels due to methylation (as per item 01) and oxygen deprivation (i.e. hydroxylation) problems (as per item 03), resulting in illnesses such as MetS (relating to hormone) or depression (relating to brain chemicals)

03 Free radical damages (due to a compromised antioxidant defense system as per item 01) on over worked cells & organs (as per item 02), will lead to a state of inflammation, oxidative stress & insulin resistance because damaged cells result in the cells' malabsorption of water/nutrients/oxygen, in particular, depressing the organ's oxygen level and impairing the organ's hydroxylation process (which requires oxygen)

01 Compromised antioxidant defense system to counter free radical attacks due to:
- A predisposition to methylation impairment arising from a methylation gene defect (i.e. **MTHFR**) combined with a low nutritional intake of vitamins & minerals (co-factors for the methylation process)
- A low intake of antioxidant food

02 Chronic stress triggers the stress response which impacts energy levels:
- Energy redirection
- Energy amplification (i.e. 5 alpha reductase enzyme activates androgenic symptoms)
- Energy over exertion (i.e. over working of either the liver or the brain)

Inability to restore chemical balance • Compromised antioxidant defense system • Overexertion due to chronic stress • Free radical damages

(B) Stress & free radical damages

Stress creates more free radical (Link 31).

Free radicals are highly reactive and unstable molecules, usually oxygen molecules, but not always. Their unstable nature is caused by having an unpaired electron. As a result of this unpaired electron, free radicals seek out and take electrons from other molecules, which oftentimes causes damage to the second molecule. When a free radical molecule does this, it is called "*oxidation*." A molecule that has had its electron "stolen" from a free radical has been "oxidized." Molecules that have been oxidized are now transformed into free radicals themselves and will seek to interact with another healthy molecule, thereby creating a vicious chain reaction of electron stealing in the body. When the body has undergone excessive oxidation, or more oxidation than can be combatted, it is said to be undergoing "*oxidative stress*". Nonetheless, at adequate amounts, free radicals help us fight infections and trigger the *inflammation or immune process* that helps repair tissue injury [excerpt from (Link 32) and with reference to (Link 33)].

But, at excessive amounts, free radicals damage the *fatty membranes* surrounding the cells (as the cells are the prime target to free radicals attacks). It is theorized here that free radicals especially target cells from organs with very high activities or vibration levels.

Hence, when there are cell damage at organs, it is not due to a random unexplainable immune system attack, a misconception (i.e. refer to Link 34). In fact, the immune process is triggered by free radicals as a protective measure during normal times. But, during chronic stress, the free radicals are the ones that cause damage to cells at organs with excessive activities or vibration level.

Organs	Very high activity level description	Free radical damage on organ cells causing impairment and diseases
Liver-gallbladder-gut	Excessive anxiety which over exerts the body systems: • Digestion, detoxification, growth/healing/immunity	Digestion problems, liver problems, immune problems
Liver-sex gland-adrenal	• Fertility	Metabolic syndrome, hormonal imbalance
Liver-pancreas-fat cells-muscles	• Metabolism	Insulin resistance (Refer section D)
Brain	Over emotional work up which over exerts the nervous system	Depression (Refer section F, G, H)

Figure B1: Free radical damage impact for selected organs

Free radicals can form in the body in a number of ways, excerpt from (Link 35):

1. ***Environmental exposure*** – Carcinogens like radiation from the sun, cigarette smoke, air and water pollution, pesticides and herbicides in the food we eat, asbestos and other nasties can cause free radical formation in our bodies.

2. ***Alcohol*** – Consumption of alcohol of any kind of any amount produces free radicals in the body.

3. ***Our bodies*** – Free radical molecules are a natural by-product of cell metabolism.

4. ***Exercise*** – While consistent moderate exercise has many positive benefits and can reduce the risk of breast cancer, excessive exercise or inconsistent but vigorous exercise uses a high amount of the body's oxygen store and as a result, generates excessive free radicals.

5. ***Fat*** – Polyunsaturated fat like that found in vegetables oils is easily oxidized in the body and can create free radicals. Substitute polyunsaturated fats with monounsaturated fat.

6. ***Obesity*** is also characterized by chronic low grade inflammation with permanently increased oxidative stress (Link 36).

7. ***Higher glucose*** increases free radicals (Link 37).

8. ***Stress*** – The chemicals cortisone and catecholamines created by mental stress can create free radicals.

(C) Problems in neutralizing free radical damages

Glutathione is the master *antioxidant/ anti-inflammatory/ detoxifier* manufactured via the *methylation* process from *glutamine* (an amino acid or protein which is abundant in our body, mostly found in muscles).

Glutathione along with other antioxidant food (i.e. vitamin C and E, blueberries, green tea, turmeric) play a crucial role in neutralising free radicals and impede their damage to cells, thus, countering oxidative stress.

An effective (i) methylation process along with sufficient (ii) glutamine levels (from protein diet intake) will ensure our antioxidant status (i.e. glutathione) is strong enough to combat the increasing free radical damages as a result of stress.

Below are problems in combatting free radicals and its associated impacts:

(i) Impaired methylation and its impact

The methylation process is involved in many critical body processes:

- Energy production
- The stress (fight-or-flight) response
- The inflammation response
- The immune response, controlling T-cell production, fighting infections and viruses and regulating the immune response
- *The production and recycling of glutathione — the body's master antioxidant*
- The repair of cells damaged by free radicals
- Genetic expression and the repair of DNA
- The detoxification of hormones, chemicals and heavy metals
- Neurotransmitters and the balancing of brain chemistry

The methylation process will be compromised (i.e. around 30%-70% inefficiency) if the body possesses some inherited *gene defects (i.e. MTHFR, MTRR, MAO, COMT)*, refer [Link 38] and [Link 39]. The inefficiency is largely expressed during stressful times.

Radical theory on MetS & Depression

A person with methylation defects easily succumbs to hormonal imbalances and illnesses when faced with stress, demonstrated as follows:

Stress level	Suppression of sex hormones to support cortisol production (cortisol steal)			Impact on body systems without methylation or MTHFR defects		Impact on body systems with methylation or MTHFR defects (30-70% inefficiency countering free radicals in times of stress)		Suppression of sex hormones to support cortisol production (cortisol steal) and depletion of sex hormones due to a weak sex gland in converting cholesterol from the liver into sex hormones		
	Progesterone level (pathway 1, 2)	Testosterone level	Estrogen level	Cortisol level	Impact on body systems	Cortisol level	Impact on body systems	Progesterone level (pathway 1, 2)	Testosterone level	Estrogen level
Baseline	1- Baseline 2- Baseline	Baseline	Baseline	Baseline	Normal	Baseline	Normal	1- Baseline 2- Baseline	Baseline	Baseline
Mid high	1- Baseline 2- Low	Low	Low	Mid high	Low suppression	High	Mid suppression (i.e. sub MetS & subfertility)	1- Low 2- Lower	Lower	Lower
High	1- Low 2- Lower	Lower	Lower	High	Mid suppression (i.e. sub MetS & subfertility)	Highest (start of adrenal fatigue, cortisol reduce)	High suppression (i.e. MetS & infertility)	1- Very low 2- Extremely Low	Extremely low	Extremely low
Higher	1- Lower 2- Very low	Very low	Very low	Higher	Mid high suppression (i.e. sub MetS & subfertility)	High	Mid suppression (i.e. but still has MetS & infertility due to extremely low testosterone)	1- Very low 2- Extremely Low	Extremely low	Extremely low
Highest	1- Very low 2- Extremely Low	Extremely low	Extremely low	Highest (start of adrenal fatigue, cortisol reduce)	High suppression (i.e. MetS & infertility)	Mid high (extreme adrenal fatigue)	Low suppression (i.e. but still has MetS & infertility due to extremely low testosterone)	1- Very low 2- Extremely Low	Extremely low	Extremely low

Figure C(i)1: Stress correlation with the hormone profile and its impact on body systems in accordance with MTHFR and methylation expression. (Refer section D(ii) on how stress impacts hormones)

As mentioned in section A(ii), when there is stress, there will be energy redirection and prioritisation of survivability over fertility, digestion, detoxification, metabolism, circulatory, mind/nervous system, growth, healing & immunity. Therefore, this is reflected in the body mechanism as cortisol increases while suppressing the above mentioned body systems.

However, when stress becomes chronic, the sex hormones are depleted to support cortisol production by the adrenal gland (termed as cortisol steal). The sex gland overworks to replenish the depleting sex hormone level while the adrenal overworks to produce cortisol to counter stress. The over activity of both the sex gland and the adrenal gland will attract free radical attacks to them. For those who do not possess methylation or MTHFR gene defects, their antioxidant defence system against free radical attacks is stronger, and hence their adrenals and sex gland only weaken when the stress level is extremely high. Hence, they can physically cope better with stress. However, for those who possess the gene defects, they cannot cope well with stress and their adrenals and sex gland start to become fatigue and produce less cortisol or sex hormone respectively faster than those who do not inherit these gene defects.

Hence, the body systems affected by chronic stress are reproduction (i.e. MetS & male fertility problems), nervous (i.e. depression), digestion, detoxification, immune, growth & healing, skeletal, circulatory, breakdown of protein/fats/carbohydrate (metabolism) [Link 40].

To minimise these genes defect expression and thus, causing inefficiency in the methylation cycle, the body needs *higher vitamins* (must have all active Bs including B8-inositol, B9-folate, B12-methylcobalamin, C) and *minerals* (zinc, magnesium) crucial for the methylation process.

It should be noted that people with MTHFR defect is unable to process folic acid (synthetic form of folate found normally in processed/packaged foods and even multivitamins that contain folic acid instead of folate). Folic acid becomes toxin in MTHFR people. Hence, will require methylated form of folate. People with MTRR defect requires higher level of B12 in its methylated form.

It should be noted that after a period of extreme stress or trauma, we need to rebuild back our body with adequate nutrition (vitamins, minerals, antioxidants, good fats, complex carbohydrate and especially protein). Our body most likely will have catabolise protein in our muscle to fuel the elevated energy requirement demanded in a hurry during the very extremely stressful period. Hence, even if the stressful event has passed, we still need to rebuild and repair the cells in the body, damaged by free radicals during the stressful phase.

(ii) Depleted glutamine level and its impact

Impact	Reason	Reference
Protein catabolisation predisposes the body to metabolism or metabolic issues	Glutamine is found abundantly in muscles	C(ii-1) C(ii-2) C(ii-3) C(ii-4)
Impaired defense against free radical damages	Depletion of antioxidant status (glutamine is the precursor to glutathione, a master antioxidant)	C(ii-1)
Impaired immunity	Glutamine is a major fuel for immune cells in the gut	C(ii-5)
Autoimmunity issues & nutrient malabsorption	Glutamine prevents leaky gut	C(ii-6)

Figure C(ii)1: Summary impact of glutamine depletion

(ii-1) Depleted protein:

Glutamine (a quick energy source) abundantly found at the muscle mass is turned into glucose (burst of energy) for quick survival reflex actions. Hence, *chronic stress will deplete glutamine (amino acid or protein) level (termed as catabolisation of protein).* We will therefore *lose muscle mass, muscle tone and deplete our master antioxidant/detoxifier-Glutathione* (because glutamine is the precursor to Glutathione). An easy noticeable symptom to alert us of protein depletion in our body is the loss of skin vibrancy (glutamine makes collagen) and knee pain (glutamine makes glucosamine, a fluid to smoothen knee movement). Thus, lower muscle mass will *slow metabolism* of fats and glucose. There is a likelihood of excess glucose and fat in our body even if our portion of food intake remains the same.

(ii-2) Excess glucose:
- Unused excess glucose is either stored in the liver or fat cells (*obesity*).
- Higher glucose increases free radicals (Link 41).

(ii-3) Excess fat:
- Unused excess fat is stored in fat cells (*obesity*).
- Excess fat along with a weak immune (as per below) to combat acne bacteria results in *acne*.

(ii-4) May lead to anxiety & trembling:

Higher GABA (a calming neurotransmitter) signalling is associated with increasing calm demeanour (i.e. calm feeling, calm movement). There are 2 pathways to provide energy for GABA signalling, that is, energy from amino acid or glucose:

- A simpler faster pathway is energy from glutamine (an amino acid/protein).
- Another pathway is from glucose via Glutamate (an excitatory amino acid based neurotransmitter) pathway. However, this pathway takes a longer time as there are many processing steps.

When the glutamine level is depleted due to catabolisation of protein as mentioned above, this may lead to anxiety and trembling movements. However, this can be countered if there is sufficient glucose intake via the Glutamate pathway, refer (Link 42) and (Link 43).

(ii-5) Impaired Immunity:
- Glutamine is the primary fuel source for the immune cells in the gut.
- Depleted glutamine impairs these cells. Hence, this will result in a *weak immunity*.

(ii-6) Leaky gut:
- Glutamine is a regulator of intestinal tight junction barriers and a depletion of this amino acid leads to rapid increases in gut permeability.
- Increased gut permeability (*leaky gut*) enables substances such as undigested food, toxins and microbes to leak through the gut wall, which may trigger *autoimmune diseases*. Refer (Link 44).
- Leaky gut /intestinal wall permeability *reduces nutrient absorption* (protein, carbohydrate, vitamin, mineral, fat). In particular, the list of amino acids which may not be adequately absorbed that impacts the methylation or hydroxylation processes are as per figure C(ii)2.

Amino acid	Methylation [Ref: C(i)]	Hydroxylation [Ref: Figure D2 and F(i-1)2]
Glutamine	✓	
Arginine	✓	✓
Proline	✓	✓
Asparagine	✓	✓
Methionine	✓	
Leucine	✓	✓
Lysine	✓	✓
Tyrosine		✓
Tryptophan	✓	✓
Valine		✓
Threonine	✓	
Serine	✓	
Alanine	✓	
Cysteine	✓	
Aspartic Acid		✓
Glutamic acid		✓
Phenylalanine		✓
Glycine		✓
Histidine		✓
Isoleucine		✓

Figure C(ii)2: Potential inadequate gut absorption of amino acids which may jeopardize the methylation and hydroxylation processes (Link 45)

In particular, some information on amino acids listed in figure C(ii)2:

Glutamine
Essential to maintain normal & steady blood sugar levels. Helps muscle strength and endurance. Gastrointestinal function; provides energy to small intestines. Precursor to Arginine.

Arginine
Plays a key role in the metabolic, immune and reparative response to trauma. In addition, it helps heal wounds/tissue repairs, release hormones, cell division and remove ammonia from the body. This amino acid is a precursor of nitric oxide, which causes blood vessel relaxation and thus, is important in the regulation of blood pressure.

Note: *Both Glutamine and Arginine become deficient in conditions of stress (i.e. trauma, critical illness). Become essential under conditions of stress and catabolic states* (Link 46).

Proline
Critical component of cartilage, aids in joint health, tendons and ligaments. Keeps heart muscle strong.

Asparagine
One of the two main excitatory neurotransmitters.

Methionine
An antioxidant. Helps in breakdown of fats and aids in reducing muscle degeneration.

Leucine
Beneficial for skin, bone and tissue wound healing.

Lysine
Component of muscle protein, and is needed in the synthesis of enzymes and hormones. It is also a precursor for L-carathine, which is essential for healthy nervous system function.

Tyrosine
Precursor of dopamine, norepinephrine and adrenaline. Increases energy, improves mental clarity and concentration, can treat some depressions. Essential for the production of important hormones like thyroxine (i.e. thyroid hormone), which plays a key role in regulating metabolism, mental health, skin health and the human growth rate.

Tryptophan
Necessary for neurotransmitter serotonin (synthesis). Effective sleep aid, due to conversion to serotonin. Reduces anxiety and some forms of depression. Treats migraine headaches. Stimulates growth hormone.

Valine
Essential for muscle development.

Threonine
Required for formation of collagen. Helps prevent fatty deposits in liver. Aids in antibodies' production.

Serine
One of the three most important glycogenic amino acids, the others being alanine and glycine. Maintains blood sugar levels, and boosts immune system. Myelin sheaths contain serine.

Alanine
Important source of energy for muscle. One of the three most important glycogenic amino acids. The primary amino acid in sugar metabolism. Boosts immune system by producing antibodies.

Cysteine, glutamic acid, glycine
These three amino acid synthesizes glutathione, the master anti-oxidant/detoxifier in the body.

Aspartate
Increases stamina and helps protect the liver; DNA and RNA metabolism; immune system function.

Phenylalanine
Beneficial for healthy nervous system. It boosts memory and learning.

Histidine
Found in high concentrations in hemoglobin. Treats anemia, has been used to treat rheumatoid arthritis.

Isoleucine
Necessary for the synthesis of hemoglobin.

Note 1: Excerpt from Link 47 which also contains detailed information of the above.

Note 2: A higher rate of protein level intake over protein loss is required to heal leaky gut.

(D) Impact of stress on the neuroendocrine functions:

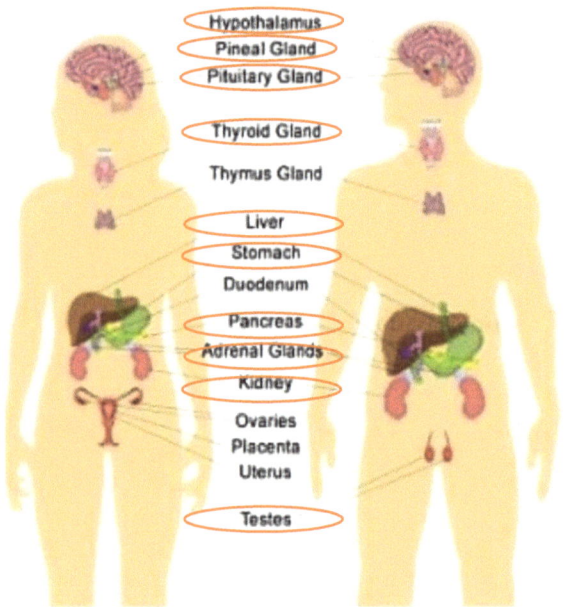

Organs in focus	Reference section
Hypothalamus	A(ii), F(i-1)
Pineal gland	F(i-1)
Pituitary gland	A(ii)
Thyroid gland	D(i-3)
Liver	D
Stomach	D(iv)
Pancreas	D(i-1), D(i-2)
Adrenal glands	A(ii), C(i), D(ii)
Kidney	D(iii)
Testes	D(ii)

Figure D1: The endocrine system image from (Link 48)

(i) Metabolic issues (insulin resistance, increasing triglycerides, protein depletion from muscles, diabetes, thyroid problems, central obesity, acne)

(i-1): Insulin resistance, increasing triglycerides, protein depletion from muscles

Chronic stress will cause the pancreas to signal the liver via glucagon hormone for more glucose (energy), and the liver will heed the order through the release of glucose to the bloodstream. Subsequently, insulin hormone from the pancreas signals the muscle to take in the glucose (*glucose uptake*) from the blood. Any unused glucose will be returned to the liver for storage as glycogen and if in excess, to fat cells (triglycerides). The unused glucose is usually due to a sedentary lifestyle or inactivity.

However, as chronic stress continues, free radicals increase, and if they are not countered by an antioxidant, the damaged membranes surrounding the liver cells will *lose its ability to transport oxygen, nutrients (i.e. amino acid, glucose, fats, vitamins & minerals) or water to the cell* (Link 49). This is when **insulin resistance** develops, where the overworked and damaged liver has difficulties transporting excess sugar or glucose out of the bloodstream and put it as storage into the liver cells. It takes a higher level of insulin (*hyperinsulinemia*) to ensure excess glucose is absorbed into the liver cells. (Link 50). Hence, **insulin resistance or insulin receptor insensitivity** *is a marker for oxidative stress, inflammation and free radical damage to the liver, in particular the liver's estrogen receptor alpha* (refer section A figure A(iii)1).

Consequently, a higher proportion of excess glucose is thus stored in fat cells (*triglycerides*) rather than as **glycogen** in the liver (hence, *higher lipogenesis* and *lower glycogen storage and synthesis*).

This leads to a higher rate of gluconeogenesis (the liver makes glucose from amino acids from muscles, from the glycerol derived from triglycerides breakdown and from other dietary sugars) because glycogen stores in the liver are low.

In short, a weakened liver due to stress would result in insulin resistance, increasing triglycerides (or obesity) and depletion of protein from our muscles.

(i-2): Diabetes

Following from the above scenario, due to the liver's increasing insulin resistance, the pancreas has to overwork to produce insulin and will eventually become fatigue. This is when *type 2 diabetes* occurs, when the body does not make enough or use the insulin well. The pancreas' over activity will attract free radical attacks to the pancreas and if the body's antioxidant defence system is weak to counter the attacks, the pancreas weakens and either makes little or no insulin, termed as *type 1 diabetes*.

(i-3): Thyroid problems

60% of the thyroid hormone thyroxine (T4) is converted to T3 in the liver prior to its distribution to target tissues. However, due to the damages sustained by the liver from free radical attacks, the liver will lose its ability to transport oxygen, nutrients or water to the cell. Hence, the thyroid has to overwork to produce more thyroid hormones for it to be absorbed by the liver due to the liver's transport problem. This is when *hyperthyroidism* occurs. The thyroid's over activity will attract free radical attacks to the thyroid and if the body's antioxidant defence system is weak to counter the attacks, the thyroid eventually weakens and makes very little of the thyroid hormone, termed as *hypothyroidism*.

(i-4): Central obesity

MetS factors such as inflammation, insulin resistance and as well as obesity lead to higher aromatization of testosterone to estradiol (Link 51), leading to decreasing testosterone level and initial increasing estradiol level. Low serum total testosterone predicts the development of central obesity in men (Link 52). [Refer to figure A5 and D(ii)1 with regards to aromatization].

(i-5): Acne

Causes	Explanation
Increasing lipids	• Free fatty acid, triglycerides (i.e. storage unit of excess fat in the body), squalene (precursor to cholesterol), cholesterol (refer iii below), cholesterol esters, wax esters and diglycerides will increase sebum secretion activity by the sebaceous gland that will promote acne. • *The level of squalene is higher in acne prone individuals* (Link 53). This is due to the backlog of squalene not being synthesized into cholesterol arising from an impaired hydroxylation process (refer iii below). • *When squalene undergoes oxidation, it produces squalene peroxide, a highly comedogenic substance and precursor to acne* (Link 54).
Decreasing antioxidant	• Another hallmark of sebum in acne patients besides squalene peroxide is a *decrease in the level of vitamin E* (refer iv below), the major sebum antioxidant (Link 55).
Androgenic	• Acne patients produce higher rates of testosterone and 5 alpha *DHT* in their skin (Link 56), and DHT spurs sebaceous gland activity. Refer A(ii) with regards to DHT.
Low immunity	• *P. Acne bacteria* has been implicated in the occurrence of acne via the induction of inflammatory mediators (Link 57) and the bacteria maybe unopposed due to low immunity stemming from *low vitamin A and D* (refer iv below).

Figure D(i-5)1: Root causes of acne

Note: Acne on forehead denotes over emotional mental stress by the overworked brain while acne on lower chin denotes over anxious stress by the overworked liver.

Practising weight loss and nutritious food intake [i.e. antioxidants, protein, phytoestrogens, low bad fat, good fat and low glycemic index (GI)] will improve insulin sensitivity, diabetes, obesity and acne:

- Liver fat content [refer D(iv)] is an important contributor to the variation in insulin clearance and could contribute to *decreased insulin clearance* in obesity (Link 58). Insulin clearance increases by weight loss (Link 59).

- ***Antioxidant has been shown to improve insulin sensitivity*** in MetS because it counters free radical damages (Link 60).

- Nevertheless, insulin resistance persists because damaged membranes surrounding cell walls are not repaired due to depleted Arginine, a protein, which is derived from Glutamine - refer section C(ii-6). Arginine plays an important role in tissue repair and wound healing. Hence, ***Arginine can improve insulin sensitivity*** (Link 61).

- Apart from exercising, a ***paleo diet focusing on a low glycemic index load along with reducing high fat milk consumption*** will help in reducing obesity and acne, as well as improving insulin resistance, refer (Link 62) and Link 63).

- Evidence is emerging that dietary ***phytoestrogens*** (i.e. soy, a plant based protein) play a ***beneficial role in obesity and diabetes.*** Nutritional intervention studies performed in animals and humans suggest that the ***ingestion of soy protein associated with isoflavones*** and ***flaxseed rich in lignans (i.e. good fat) improves glucose control and insulin resistance*** (Link 64). (Note: Extensive scientific research has shown no effects of soy protein or isoflavone intake on testosterone or estrogen levels in men).

Hydroxylation

- ***Without adequate oxygen transported into the endocrine organs, this impairs the hydroxylation process in the endocrine organs because hydroxylation process requires oxygen.*** Hydroxylation is an ***oxidation*** reaction through conversion of a hydrogen to a hydroxyl group via addition of oxygen (Link 65).

- Hydroxylation reactions play a very important role in the synthesis of cholesterol from squalene, in the conversion of cholesterol into steroid hormones [sex hormones, cortisol, vitamin d (a type of hormone) and other hormones] and in the conversion of cholesterol to bile salts (Link 66).

- Hydroxylation is an oxidation reaction that is involved in the liver's phase 1 detoxification process.

- Thus, impairment in the hydroxylation processes leads to:

  - Hormonal imbalance due to inadequate conversion of cholesterol into sex hormones by the sex gland.

  - Weak cholesterol profile due to inadequate synthesis of cholesterol from squalene by the liver (high ldl), inadequate conversion of cholesterol into bile salts by the liver (low hdl) and inadequate conversion of cholesterol into steroid hormones by the sex gland and the adrenal gland (high total cholesterol).

  - Lowered production of bile acid causing bile sluggishness due to inadequate conversion of cholesterol into bile salts by the liver.

  - Impairment in the liver's phase 1 detoxification process.

  Note: Refer below ii-v for more information.

Figure D2: Hydroxylation

(ii) Hormonal imbalance (low sex drive, fertility issues, sexual dysfunction, sperm production problems, feminization)

Worries/ anxieties/ fears trigger the adrenal gland to produce cortisol hormone to combat the stress. However, as stress increases, the body favours the production of cortisol and suppresses the production of sex hormones (both cortisol and sex hormones share the same base ingredient, pregnenolone), termed as the ***cortisol steal*** [refer to A(ii) which talks about energy redirection]. Very little of the pregnenolone will be transformed into progesterone, testosterone and thereafter estrogen because pregnenolone is redirected to support cortisol level. Initially, the level of testosterone maybe depleting but is still at an adequate level. Low testosterone can directly affect male fertility by causing a decrease in sperm production. It indirectly affects fertility by reducing his sex drive and causing ***erectile dysfunction***.

But, if the stress is excessive, the sex gland will be overworked (attracting free radical attacks undefended by a weak methylation process resulting in free radical damages, inflammation and oxidative stress, leading to an impaired hydroxylation process of the sex gland) in replenishing the depleting sex hormones. Thus, over time, there will be ***hormonal imbalances*** leading to ***male subfertility***. Eventually, there will be *low levels of the sex hormones testosterone*, ***as well as progesterone and*** *estrogen* [refer to figure C(i)1 which demonstrates the depletion of sex hormones to support cortisol production]. Low sex hormones would result in a ***low sex drive***.

The liver would be overworked (attracting free radical attacks undefended by a weak methylation process resulting in free radical damages to ERα, inflammation and oxidative stress, leading to an impaired hydroxylation process of the liver) in producing cholesterol from squalene, where the cholesterol is then transformed to pregnenolone by either the adrenal or the sex gland. The liver makes 80% of the cholesterol in the body. Cholesterol is first transformed into pregnenolone which is the precursor to the sex hormones (progesterone, testosterone and thereafter estrogen), cortisol, vitamin D and other hormones (collectively known as steroid hormones).

The low sex hormones are not adequately replenished back to baseline levels ***due to an inadequate synthesis of cholesterol from squalene by the liver and inadequate conversion of cholesterol into sex hormones by the sex gland arising from an impaired hydroxylation process (refer figure D2).***

Features	Explanation
Luteinizing hormone (LH) pulsation increases Follicle-stimulating hormone (FSH) pulsation increases	The hypothalamus detected low testosterone level and thus, the pituitary increases LH and FSH pulsation. Thereafter, LH stimulates the release of testosterone from Leydig cells of the testes while FSH stimulates sperm production from Sertoli cells of the testes
Increasing aromatization rate Decreasing testosterone level Initial increasing estradiol level Decreasing T/E ratio which results in feminization	However, testosterone is ***aromatised*** to estradiol, resulting in decreasing testosterone (T) and initial increasing estradiol (E) levels. Thus, ***T/E ratio is decreasing*** Note: The aromatization rate can be increased due to metabolic syndrome (MetS) factors such as obesity, insulin resistance, inflammation and consumption of alcohol while the rate can be decreased by prolactin and anti-Mullerian hormone. [Refer to (Link 67) , (Link 68) and figure A5 with regards to aromatization]
Sexual dysfunction, fertility issues, sperm production problems, low sex drive	Low testosterone level leads to sexual dysfunction, fertility issues, sperm production problems and low sex drive (refer Link 69)

Figure D(ii)1: The features above correlates with the article (Link 70) entitled "Psychological stress primarily lowers serum total testosterone level with secondary rise in serum LH and FSH levels altering seminal quality"

Therefore, there is a high probability of ***sexual dysfunction, infertility***, ***low sperm production and low sex drive*** due to the low testosterone level. The initial increasing estradiol combined with decreasing testosterone level will lead to the feminization of men (i.e. breast tissue growth). *If the chronic stress continues, the estrogen level will eventually be decreased as well.*

However, even after the chronic stress event has passed and there is less demand for cortisol, an *impaired hydroxylation process will cause the state of low progesterone, testosterone and estrogen to persist, prolonging the Metabolic syndrome & infertility.*

Protein intake to improve liver, brain, hormonal balance & fertility:
- *Adequate level of estrogen provides protection against oxidative stress in both the liver's mitochondria and the brain's mitochondria through the up-regulation of antioxidant genes* (i.e. glutathione peroxidase). However, estrogen supplementation may have tumour promotion and feminizing properties, hence, *phytoestrogens (i.e. soy) are a good alternative in protecting the liver and the brain* (Link 71) for they do not possess tumour promotion and feminizing properties. Nonetheless, phytoestrogens should be used in moderation. Refer article (Link 72) on the pros & cons of phytoestrogen. *There is some evidence that the intake of plant sourced proteins and in particular, soy protein associated with isoflavones may prevent the onset of risk factors associated with metabolic syndrome* (Link 73). Soy also reduces 5 alpha reductase (Link 74).

- *Repairing the liver cell walls via Arginine (protein)* will improve nutrient, water, oxygen intake and thus, hormonal balance (Link 75).

Note:
- Though there are studies that state that testosterone therapy can help in improving MetS in men, for example, (Link 76) and (Link 77), however, caution should be undertaken as external application of testosterone can reduce sperm production and thus fertility (Link 78).

(iii) **Weak cholesterol profile (cholesterol plagues, cardiovascular problems, high blood pressure, kidney problems)**

The depleted sex hormone levels *trigger higher cholesterol production* because the body thinks it needs more cholesterol to make new sex hormones in the body. However, the sex gland and the adrenal gland's inadequate conversion of cholesterol into steroid hormones (i.e. sex hormones, cortisol, vitamin D and other hormones) arising from an impaired hydroxylation process will cause a backlog of untransformed cholesterol, leading to a state of increasing total cholesterol level.

The impaired hydroxylation process also causes the liver's inadequate synthesis of cholesterol from squalene (a precursor to cholesterol), leading to a backlog of increasing untransformed squalene. It should be noted that squalene, either biosynthesized or dietary, is secreted into very low density lipoproteins (VLDL) and low density lipoproteins (LDL) and distributed to various tissues. Skin is also a biosynthetic tissue for squalene to provide the large quantities found in the sebaceous gland (Link 79).

It should be noted that cholesterol is secreted via the liver's bile. Hence, a lowered bile movement due to hydroxylation problem (refer section iv below) would mean, less cholesterol is excreted out (*lesser cholesterol removal*). Additionally, a sluggish bile leads to malabsorption of fat soluble vitamin D and E that reduces production of HDL from the intestines (Link 80).

Therefore, an impaired hydroxylation process will lead to a weak cholesterol profile (i.e. an increasing total cholesterol level, an increasing squalene level followed by an increasing VLDL and LDL level along with a decreasing HDL cholesterol level).

LDL cholesterol is the raw material of cholesterol plagues. As this cholesterol plague builds up along artery walls, it slowly blocks the blood flow in the arteries (*increasing blood pressure*). A cholesterol plague can suddenly rupture. The sudden blood clot that forms over the rupture then causes a heart attack or stroke (*cardiovascular problems*) (Link 81).

Increasing blood pressure as mentioned above together with higher fat & sugar in the blood [refer D(i-1)] can place a great strain on the kidneys due to its role as the blood filtering units of the body. Hence, the ***kidneys are prone to problems*** with blood circulation and blood vessels (Link 82).

Increasing fibre, soy & any other protein intake together with limiting excessive carbohydrate intake will improve cholesterol, blood pressure levels and prevent cardiovascular & kidney problems:

- *Arginine (protein) can improve cholesterol* through improvement in bile flow through its function of blood vessel relaxation [refer to section C(ii-6)], (Link 83).

- An article (Link 84) states that ***high LDL cholesterol actually signifies a lack of tryptophan (protein from the diet).***

- Several studies in humans and animals have shown that ***soy isoflavones (protein) reduce plasma total cholesterol and LDL cholesterol*** (Link 85). Protein is crucial in repairing damaged cell walls, thus, improving the hydroxylation process and preventing a backlog of cholesterol.

- Limiting excessive carbohydrate intake as higher glucose increases free radicals that damage cell walls (Link 86).

- Dietary intake of fibre can also prevent the re-absorption of cholesterol before recycling back into the body, thus, helping in decreasing excessive level of cholesterol.

According to (Link 87);

- Testosterone replacement replaces dyslipidemia (weak cholesterol) in men.
    - Androgen replacement can decrease blood serum levels of cholesterol and LDL via enhancing liver *cholesterol uptake* and via suppressing *cholesterol removal* which in turn increases liver cholesterol accumulation.
    - Increased testosterone will lead to increased *cholesterol synthesis* but thereafter, the cholesterol level will revert back to baseline level.

Note:

- In the author's opinion, artificially increasing the testosterone level will signal to the body to become more androgenic, and therefore, the body will think that it is facing a threat [do refer to A(ii) with regards to energy redirection & amplification]. Thereafter, the body will increase cholesterol synthesis and uptake in the liver and reduce cholesterol removal in the liver in order to accumulate cholesterol to make cortisol hormone to face the threat/anxious stress.

(iv) <u>**Lowered bile movement or bile sluggishness (bad bacteria build up, gut issues, toxin build up, liver fat, vision problems, weak immunity, infertility, inflammation, skin health issues, bruising)**</u>

Inadequate conversion of cholesterol into bile salts arising from an impaired hydroxylation process will impair the gut environment as follows:

- ***Bad bacteria build up***. Gut bacteria helps make serotonin and dopamine in the gut (<u>Link 88</u>). But, a non-hospitable gut environment where there is increasing bad bacteria over good bacteria will jeopardise the production of serotonin & dopamine in the gut. As serotonin & dopamine in the gut control gut motility, this will lead to a low gut motility (***constipation***) problem.

- This in turn will lead to slow elimination of waste products (***toxin build up***) and many ***gut issues***- diarrhoea, trapped gas, bad-smelling gas, stomach cramps, erratic bowel movement and pale-coloured stools.

- ***Lower metabolism or digestion of fats for energy*** *(lowered lipolysis)*, hence, accumulation of liver fat *(increasing lipid uptake)*, also termed as fatty liver. If the fat accumulation at the liver progresses, this will lead to an irreversible ***non-alcoholic fatty liver disease*** (NAFLD) and finally to ***cirrhosis*** (scar tissue at the liver).

- *Malabsorption of fat soluble vitamins such as A, D, E, K.*

Low vitamin	Impact
A	*Impair vision, low immunity*
D	*Low immunity, infertility*
E	*Reduce antioxidant to neutralize free radicals & thus, higher inflammation, Skin health impairment*
K	*Easy bruising, reduced blood clotting*

Figure D(iv)1: Low vitamin A, D, E, K level and its impact

As per article (<u>Link 89</u>), some natural ways to improve bile flow are:
- Warm water with the juice of one lemon in the morning to cleanse the liver
- Liver friendly foods such as radish, leeks, asparagus, celery and carrots
- Eliminate even good fats and oils from the diet for a period of time to allow your liver a rest from digesting fats
- Avoid sugary and processed foods
- Eat cultured vegetables packed with probiotics

(v) <u>**Impaired detoxification (toxin build up, imbalance hormone & neurotransmitter level)**</u>
The inefficiency in hydroxylation, an oxidation reaction [as mentioned in figure D2: hydroxylation above] will adversely impact the liver's phase 1 detoxification process. Along with the inefficiency in methylation [as mentioned in C(i)] which adversely impacts the liver's phase 2 detoxification process, ***the liver's total detoxification process is greatly impaired, leading to a build-up of toxins in the body and an imbalance hormone and neurotransmitter level.***

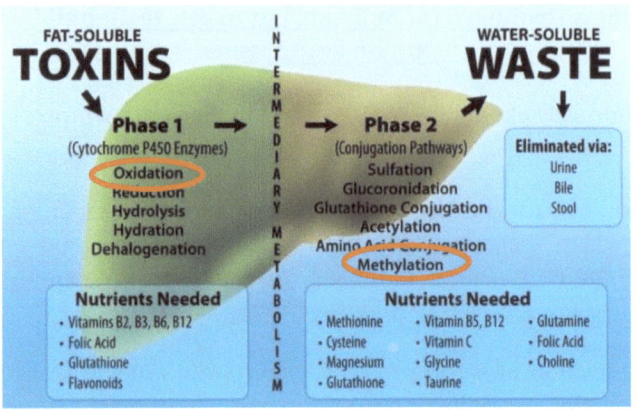

Toxins:
- Metabolic end products (i.e. hormones, neurotransmitters)
- Contaminants/pollutants
- Insecticides
- Pesticides
- Food additives
- Drugs
- Alcohol
- Micro-organisms

Figure D(v)1: Liver phase 1 and 2 detoxification (Link 90)

The nutrients needed for effective phase 1 liver detoxification are:
- vitamin Bs (B2, B3, B6, B9-folate, B12)
- antioxidant (glutathione) and
- flavonoids (naturally occurring plant pigments thought to provide health benefits through cell signalling pathways and antioxidant effects)

The nutrients needed for effective phase 2 liver detoxification are:
- protein (methionine, cysteine, glycine, taurine, glutamine)
- mineral (magnesium)
- antioxidant (glutathione)
- vitamin Bs (B5, B9-folate, B12) and C
- vitamin like (choline)

Hence, the diet or supplements should incorporate the above nutrients for effective detoxification.

Section D's reference on liver functions:
(Link 91), (Link 92), (Link 93), (Link 94), (Link 95), (Link 96), (Link 97), (Link 98), (Link 99)

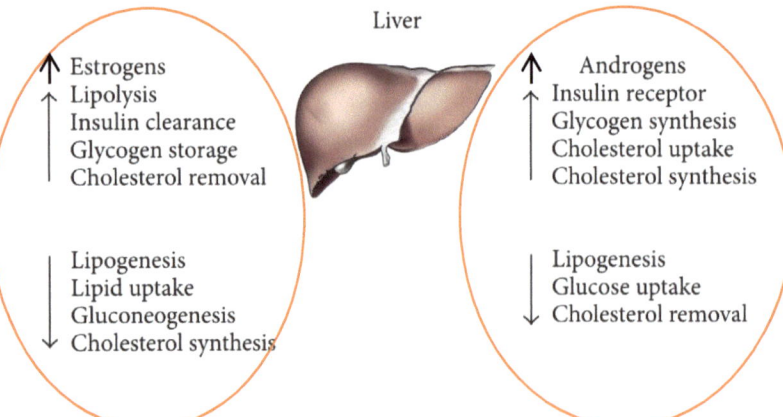

Figure D3: Items highlighted in orange under this section D is in line with this article's (Link 99) representation of metabolic effects of estrogens and androgens on regulation of lipid, glucose, and cholesterol in the liver. However, (Link 99) depicts an increasing estrogen and androgen level impact while this section D demonstrates a decreasing estrogen and androgen level impact on lipid, glucose and cholesterol in the liver.

(E) Impact of nutrition to prevent or heal from a neuroendocrine imbalance

Based on issues or root causes listed in section A, B, C, D, F and G, the table below (figure E1) provides ways to prevent or heal from a neuroendocrine imbalance through initial observatory symptoms. After which, a specific test for imbalances for a targeted organ can be undertaken and hence, to apply the correct treatment to rebalance the body.

Root cause mitigation via:	Ref.	Example	Ensuring adequacy via:	Symptoms observation if unmitigated	Test options for imbalances	Where to test	Affected organs
Higher antioxidant food to combat free radicals and prevent oxidative stress	B C	Blue berries, green tea, curcumin	Antioxidant supplement	Low energy, skin and hair issues	Oxidative stress & glutathione Cholesterol or insulin test as their increases are due to free radical damages unprotected by decreasing antioxidant	Precision analytical General practitioner	Whole body
Higher anti-inflammatory food to counter 5 alpha reductase that leads to an inflammatory & androgenic state, heal cell membrane and prevent cancer	A(ii) B C(i)	Fatty fish	Fish oil with EPA/DHA, flaxseed oil, vitamin D3, green tea, zinc, soy	Receding hairline and excessive hair growth (hirsutism) i.e. facial hair, severe acne	Inflammatory markers (i.e. AA/EPA) test	Nutripath	Whole body
Higher vitamins (must have all active Bs including B8-inositol, B9-folate, B12-methylcobalamin, C) and minerals zinc, magnesium. These vitamins/minerals are crucial for methylation [that impacts energy production; the stress/ inflammation/ immune response; antioxidant status; DNA or cell repair (i.e. prevent cancer); detoxification of hormones & chemicals; rebalancing of neurotransmitters] Vitamins A, D, E, K crucial for growth/healing & immunity	C(i)	Rainbow colour of vegetables/ fruits, in particular focusing on those containing vitamin Bs, C,A,D,E,K and mineral zinc, magnesium	Multivitamin & mineral containing the specified nutrients	Skin issues & inflammation (low vitamin E); infertility (low vitamin D); easy bruising (low vitamin K) and easily catch infection/cold due to lowered immunity (low vitamin C, D) and blur vision (low vitamin A) Observation whether there is lesser energy level or unable to cope feeling/ moodiness from low vitamin Bs	Vitamin and mineral test Basic organic acid test (B6, B12) Methylation test (**MTHFR**, MTRR, MAO, COMT)	Spectracell Precision Analytical Nutripath	Whole body

Root cause mitigation via:	Ref.	Example	Ensuring adequacy via:	Symptoms observation if unmitigated	Test options for imbalances	Where to test	Affected organs
Higher protein to repair damaged cells by free radicals (i.e. damaged liver cells leading to high LDL & low HDL cholesterol) and counter effects of protein catabolisation [i.e. knee pain, loss of skin vibrancy, depletion of master antioxidant (glutathione), loss of muscle mass, slowing of metabolism that promotes obesity/ acne, impaired immunity, anxiety and leaky gut (related to autoimmunity & nutrient malabsorption)]	D(iii) C(ii)	Soya, fish, meat, eggs, almond & walnut (contains Arginine)	Supplements i.e. protein powder or l-glutamine & arginine mostly used by fitness people. Note: Nonetheless, glutamine is not safe for mentally weak people with brains which have high neuronal activity (i.e. high glutamate) (Link 100)	Observation of loss of muscle tone, easily gain weight, acne, knee pain, loss of skin vibrancy, allergies and easily catch cold/infections Body mass index(BMI) in the correct range but Body fat percentage (BF%) very high High LDL & low HDL cholesterol	Amino acid test Leaky gut test Body Mass Index (BMI) and Body fat % Cholesterol test	Spectracell Nutripath Weighing machine with BMI and body fat % measurement General practitioner	Whole body
Plenty of water to facilitate hydroxylation process	D(i)	Water	8-10 glasses of water	If well hydrated, urine is clear with a tinge of yellow	Simple skin pinch test to test skin suppleness	N/A	Whole body
Lower bad fatty food to prevent excess fat accumulation & acne	D(i-1) D(i-4) D(i-5)	Avoid fried food and minimise trans-fat & saturated fat food	Moderate strength and cardio exercise for at least 30 mins.	Observation of bulging tummy, acne	Body fat %	Weighing machine with body fat % measurement	Whole body
Adequate calorie intake to prevent trembling/ anxiety	C(ii-4)	Complex carbohydrate such as sweet potato, oats	Food diary	Observation of trembling movements	Body mass index (BMI)	Weighing machine with BMI measurement	Whole body
Higher fibre rich food to reduce cholesterol/ artery plaque/ cardiovascular/ high blood pressure/ kidney/ acne problems	D(iii) D(i-5)	Oats	Fibre powder	Observation of oily face, acne Headaches and shortness of breath	Cholesterol test Blood pressure test	General practitioner General practitioner	Liver & kidney
Lower simple carbohydrate that quickly turns into glucose to prevent excess unused glucose and increasing accumulation in fat cells (triglycerides), insulin resistance, diabetes & acne	D(i-1) D(i-2) D(i-4) D(i-5)	Avoid package or processed food (i.e. white rice, pasta, noodles, pastries, biscuits, white bread), sugary food	Moderate strength and cardio exercise for at least 30 mins	Easily gain weight around waist, acne	Insulin test	General practitioner	Liver, pancreas

Radical theory on MetS & Depression

Root cause mitigation via:	Ref.	Example	Ensuring adequacy via:	Symptoms observation if unmitigated	Test options for imbalances	Where to test	Affected organs
Higher liver support to boost up liver's role in energy management, hormonal balancing, cholesterol management, detoxification (i.e. toxins, excess hormones & neurotransmitters), bile production and prevention of liver fats accumulation	D	Citrus fruits (helps in liver cleansing), garlic (helps in detoxifying), almond & walnut (high in arginine to repair liver)	Milk thistle supplement Arginine supplement Epsom salt bath Sauna	Observation of central obesity, oily skin, acne, bruising, skin ill health, inflammation, mood issues, sexual dysfunction, infertility, gut/ immunity & vision issues	Phase 1 Liver test or Liver test Hair mineral analysis of heavy metals	Precision Analytical Nutripath Nutripath	Liver
Higher adrenal support to boost up adrenal gland and to prevent cortisol dysregulation	C(i), D(ii)	Holy basil tea to calm the adrenals	Rhodiola rosea/ ashwagandha/ licorice root supplement	Feeling of being overwhelmed	Cortisol test	Precision Analytical	Adrenal
Higher rebalancing of sex hormones to avoid hormone imbalance, low sex hormones, low sex drive, fertility issues, sperm problems and sexual dysfunction	D(ii)	Protein & antioxidant food	Protein & antioxidant supplement	Low sex drive, fertility issues, sexual dysfunction	Sex hormone test	Precision Analytical	Sex gland
Higher probiotic to improve gut good bacteria and prevent gut issues	D(iv)	Yoghurt, kombucha, kefir, kimchi	Probiotic supplement	Observation of gut issues, constipation	Stool analysis test	Nutripath	Stomach
Higher thyroid support to boost up thyroid and prevent hyperthyroidism and hypothyroidism	D(i-3)	Brazil/ macadamia/ hazel nuts	Thyroid support supplement (i.e. zinc, vitamin A,D,E,K,B complex, C, omega 3 fats)	Hoarse voice Hyperthyroidism or hypothyroidism symptoms	Thyroid test	Nutripath	Thyroid
Higher stress relieving techniques to avoid depression, anxiety, BPD and other mental health problems	F,G, H,I,J	Meditation and mindful-ness techniques, deep breathing, gentle exercises like yoga	Journaling, talk therapy	Observation of prolong worried/sad/ angry demeanour, brain fog	Cortisol test Basic neuro-transmitter test Advance neuro-transmitter test	Precision Analytical Precision Analytical Nutripath	Adrenal Brain Brain

Figure E1: Impact of nutrition to prevent or heal from a neuroendocrine imbalance

Note 1:
To refer to nutritional guidelines and naturopathic or nutritional practitioners for more information on the types of food/supplements to address the concerned areas according to your body chemistry.

Note 2: Links of where to tests:
- Dutch plus test from Precision analytical (Link 101)
- Vitamin, mineral, amino acid test from Spectracell (Link 102)
- Functional tests listed above from Nutripath (Link 103)

(F) Depression & Neurotransmitters

(i) Neurotransmitters

Neurotransmitter is a type of chemical messenger which transmits signals across a chemical synapse, from one neuron to another target neuron, muscle cell or gland cell. Here, the study is confined to the study of 5 key neurotransmitters listed below because they appear to adequately explain depression (i.e. BPD/borderline, dysthymia, bipolar and major depression).

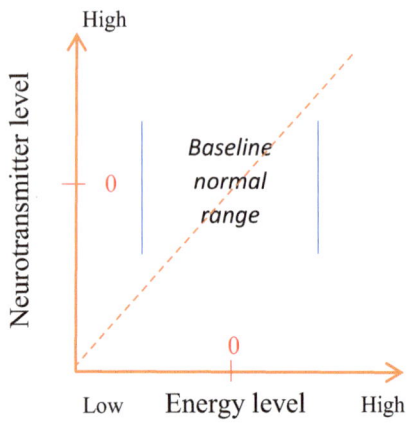

Examples of excitatory neurotransmitters are glutamate, dopamine, and serotonin.

This means, the higher the level of this neurotransmitter, it signals the cell to be more excited/vibrating (high energy level). When the cell is too excited, it is neurotoxic.

When the cell vibrates only minimally or nil vibration (too low level of neurotransmitter signalling), the cell does not express its role.

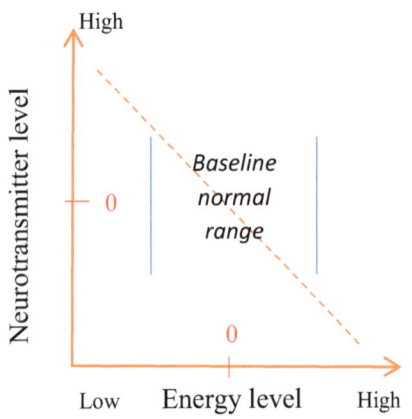

Example of an inhibitory neurotransmitter is GABA.

This means, the higher the level of this neurotransmitter, it signals the cell to be more inhibiting/less vibration (less energy level). When the cell is too inhibited, the cell vibrates only minimally or nil vibration, thus, the cell does not express its role.

On the other extreme end, too low level of this neurotransmitter will cause excitement to the cell.

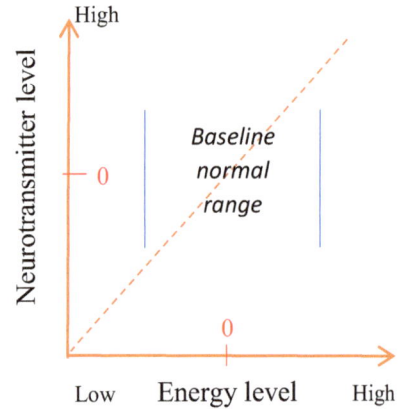

Example of a suppress inhibitory neurotransmitter is oxytocin.

This means, the higher the level of this neurotransmitter, it suppresses inhibiting cell actions (high energy level) while the lower the level, the less suppression towards inhibiting cell actions.

Figure F(i)1: Neurotransmitter charts. The combination of excitatory, inhibitory and suppress inhibitory neurotransmitter levels that accumulatively falls within the baseline normal range denotes a mentally healthy person. Health is not found at the extreme ends of the neurotransmitter level.

(i-1) Emotional mental stress, neurotransmitter over signalling, free radical attacks to brain, depression

Emotional mental stress is bad for the brain. For example, a breakup will cause one to feel frustrated (low end of the normal range for serotonin) and anxious (low end of the normal range for GABA). Then, rumination over the loss of a relationship will lead to over signalling of glutamate (learning, perception & memory intensity to discover the cause of break up), dopamine (to recover the broken relationship) and oxytocin (overwhelmed with relationship rejection) [refer section F(ii) on neurotransmitter spectrum of emotions & functions]. *Over signalling of excitatory neurotransmitter* (i.e. dopamine, glutamate) and '*suppress inhibitory neurotransmitter*' (i.e. oxytocin), will *attract free radical attacks to the over vibrating/over excited brain, leading to free radical damages, inflammation and oxidative stress.*

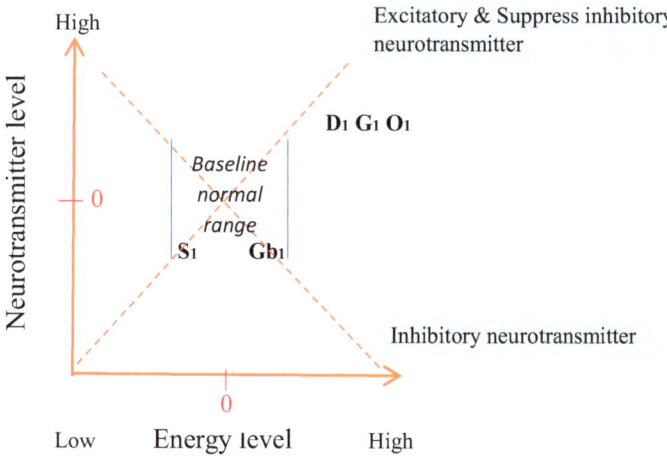

Figure F(i-1)1: Combined neurotransmitter chart – Start of mental stress

Thereafter, the damaged membranes surrounding the brain cells will *lose its ability to transport oxygen, nutrients or water* to the cell. This is when insulin resistance develops, where the brain has difficulty transporting glucose into its cells and thus, it takes more insulin hormone to ensure glucose absorption into the brain (*brain insulin resistance*). Brain insulin resistance deteriorates cognition by altering the topology of brain networks (Link 104).

Hydroxylation & oxygen deprivation in the brain

Crucially, the *hydroxylation process of the brain is impaired* as oxygen is required for hydroxylation (an oxidation process), leading to the brain's:

- Inefficient synthesis of cholesterol in the brain, impairing learning (Link 105)
- Inefficient cholesterol turnover and excretion from the brain via the bile acid pathway, leading to high cholesterol in the brain. Maybe associated with formation of beta-amyloid plaques seen in Alzheimer's disease (Link 105 and Link 106)
- Inefficient neurotransmitter production (i.e. serotonin, dopamine), leading to the brain's neurotransmitter imbalance

Additionally, a state of depressed oxygen level in the brain also lowers the neurotransmitter production of GABA, glutamate and oxytocin, compounding the brain's neurotransmitter imbalance (Link 107).

Figure F(i-1)2: Hydroxylation and oxygen deprivation in the brain

A brain environment with *low oxygen level will reduce tryptophan hydrolase production and tyrosine hydrolase production* at the hypothalamus and consequently, *greatly depresses the availability of serotonin and dopamine respectively.* Meanwhile, the depressed oxygen level in the brain also reduces GABA, glutamate and oxytocin. Accumulatively, there is more brain inhibiting energy over excitatory energy. *This is when major depression with anxiety develops.*

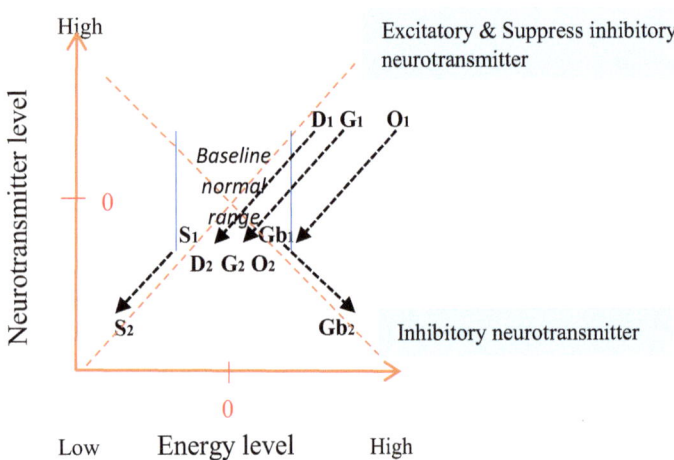

Figure F(i-1)3: Combined neurotransmitter chart – Major depression with anxiety

It should be noted that disturbed serotonin availability can lead to carbohydrate craving, because carbohydrate-rich diet triggers insulin response to enhance bioavailability of tryptophan in the central nervous system (Link 108).

Serotonin is a precursor to melatonin (sleep hormone). Within the pineal gland, serotonin is acetylated and then methylated to yield melatonin. Therefore, with the depressed level of serotonin as mentioned above, melatonin level greatly drops, leading to sleep problems or insomnia.

Fortunately, *antioxidant action* (i.e. vitamin E) restores tryptophan hydrolase and serotonin levels in the hypothalamus (Link 109). Hence, a person with a good glutathione level (master detoxifier & antioxidant), as part of the methylation process will be *protected against depression.*

Natural healing

Brain cells can be renewed via a process called *neurogenesis*, which include undertaking activities as per below. It should be noted that stress dampens neurogenesis (Link 110).

- Indulge in uplifting and interesting hobbies & exercises with friends (increase the low serotonin level) and distraction from rumination over problem (lower the high glutamate, high oxytocin and high dopamine level).
- Relax/ pray/ meditate/ mindfulness techniques (increase the low GABA level, decrease the high dopamine level).
- Eat antioxidant food, especially the 4 outstanding food to reduce oxidative stress:

    blueberries, omega 3 fatty acid, green tea, curcumin (Link 111).

Conventional healing

Fortunately, there is potential antioxidant action of antidepressants to counter oxidative damage which contributes to depression (Link 112).

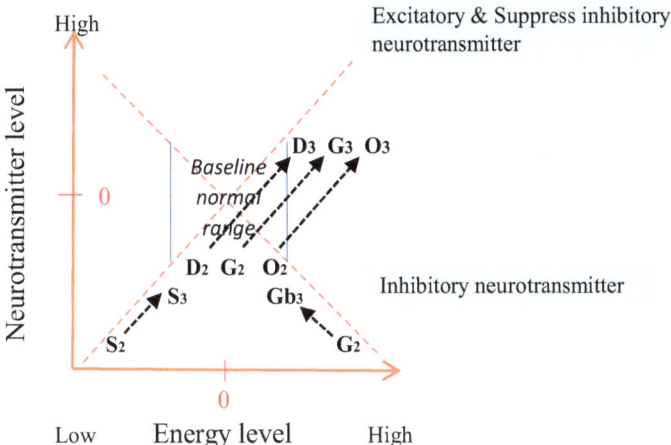

Figure F(i-1)4: Combined neurotransmitter chart – Borderline depression or BPD

Note:

Neurogenesis actions or antidepressant intake will increase all neurotransmitters.

Though there is no more symptoms of major depression and accumulatively, the inhibitory and excitatory energy of the brain is in equilibrium, nonetheless, dopamine, glutamate and oxytocin are still at borderline high levels while serotonin and GABA are at borderline low levels because the brain is not rebalanced to baseline range due to ineffective methylation.

This represents Borderline depression or Borderline Personality Disorder (BPD), a form of resistant depression.

(i-2) Chronic emotional mental stress, brain neurotoxin, resistant depression

Following from the above example, if rumination over the relationship breakup continues, this will lead to a state of *chronic emotional mental stress*, with extreme over signalling of excitatory neurotransmitter (i.e. dopamine, glutamate) and 'suppress inhibitory neurotransmitter' (i.e. oxytocin). Thereafter, target cells become extremely excited which leads to accumulation of *neurotoxin* in the brain. If we have a genetic methylation defect, our brain will be ineffective in detoxing this neurotoxin. Hence, the *depression becomes resistant* and glutamate, dopamine, oxytocin and estrogen receptor beta (ERβ) receptors are damaged:

Overstimulation of glutamate receptors cause neurodegeneration and neuronal damage (*impairing learning, perception and memory*) through a process called *excitotoxicity*. Glutamate excitotoxicity triggered by overstimulation of glutamate receptors also contributes to intracellular oxidative stress. Proximal glial cells use a cystine/glutamate antiporter (xCT) to transport cystine into the cell and glutamate out. Excessive extracellular glutamate concentrations reverse xCT, so glial cells no longer have enough cystine to synthesize glutathione (GSH), an antioxidant. Lack of GSH leads to more reactive oxygen species (ROSs) or free radicals that damage and kill the glial cell, which then cannot reuptake and process extracellular glutamate [excerpt from (Link 113)].

Additionally, unopposed increasing free radicals due to a weak antioxidant defence system (controlled by the methylation process) will lead to damages to dopamine & oxytocin receptors and estrogen receptor beta (ERβ), where colocalisation of ERβ is found in oxytocin-containing cells (Link 114).

The brain ERβ damages is in line with section A figure A(iii)2/ 3/ 4 and 5.

Damaged oxytocin receptors impair modulation of a variety of behaviours, including stress and anxiety, social memory and recognition, sexual and aggressive behaviours, bonding (affiliation) and maternal behaviour.

Abnormal dopamine receptor signalling and dopaminergic nerve function impairs many neurological processes, including motivation, pleasure, cognition, memory, learning, and fine motor control, as well as modulation of neuroendocrine signalling [excerpt from (Link 115)].

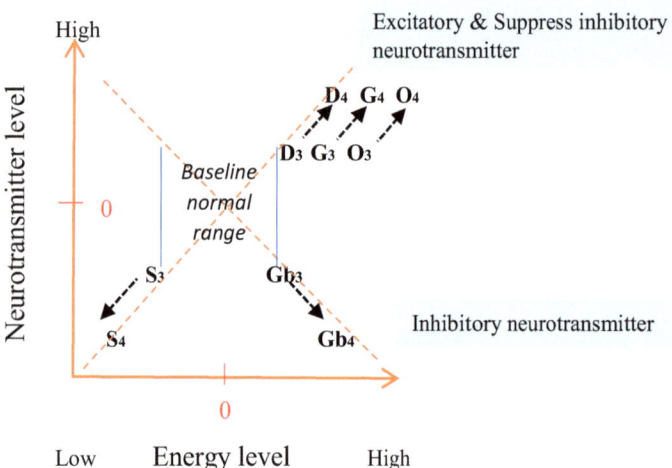

Figure F(i-2)1: Combined neurotransmitter chart – BPD splitting

Note:

Borderline depression or BPD individuals cannot cope well with stress, where any frustration or anxiety triggers will amplify serotonin and GABA to even lower levels beyond the baseline normal range while amplifying dopamine, glutamate and oxytocin to even higher levels beyond the baseline normal range.

The above adequately explains the splitting behaviour associated with BPD where they fluctuate between normalcy and extreme emotions.

Apart from MTHFR and MTRR [refer C(i)], the COMT and MAO-A genes are crucial in the methylation actions to rebalance neurotransmitters back to baseline levels.

During major depression, the MAO-A is sped up/elevated (Link 116). In particular, there is an article linking between *elevated MAO-A activity (which decreases serotonin levels) with Borderline Personality Disorder (BPD)* (Link 117). Low serotonin decreases our feeling of wellbeing. Treatment should target in providing co-factors required for neurotransmitter synthesis and providing precursors for serotonin such as vitamin B-6 and 5-HTP (Link 118).

Though dopamine level is decreased as well due to the elevated MAO-A, the reduction is likely to be lesser compared with the *increases in stress chemicals* levels such as dopamine, adrenaline and noradrenaline arising from a *decrease in COMT activity.* Excess stress chemicals make us feel unable to cope even with a small stressor. Treatment should target supplementing with magnesium, vitamin C and Bs [(Link 119) and (Link 120)].

This is substantiated by the article (Link 121) which demonstrates that *the Met158 allele encoding for the COMT with low enzymatic efficiency was found to be over-represented in Borderline Personality Disorder, possibly resulting in excessive synaptic dopaminergic activity and ultimately affecting externalizing behaviours, such as impulsivity and aggressiveness.*

In another article, it highlights the *impact of childhood trauma and adverse life events (trauma load)* on a person with COMT Met allele, predisposing the individual to be at risk for depression. Conversely, a trauma on a person with COMT Val allele creates resilience instead (Link 122).

Trauma and chronic stress lead to *body-wide DNA methylation changes,* predisposing a person to mental and physical illness. The methylation changes *may pass down through generations* (Link 123).

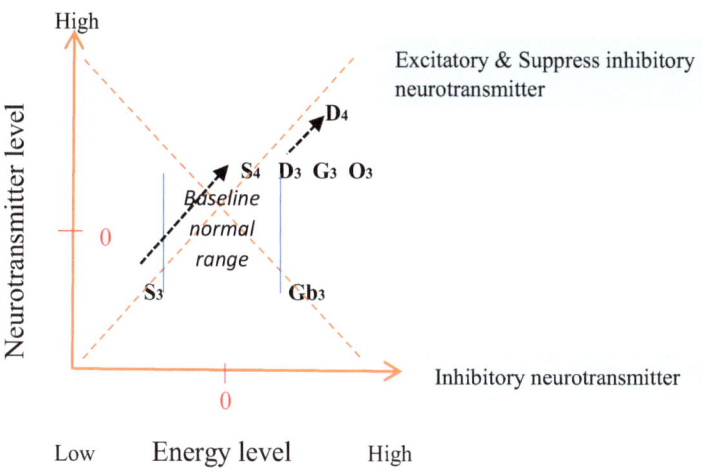

Figure F(i-2)2: Combined neurotransmitter chart – Bipolar (hypomania or mania phase)

Note:

A borderline depression [as per F(i-1)4] combined with further excessive protein intake (i.e. tryptophan and tyrosine which are dietary precursors to serotonin and dopamine respectively), can further elevate serotonin (S_3 to S_4) and dopamine (D_3 to D_4) to higher levels.

As such, dopamine would be at an extremely high level alongside high levels of glutamate and oxytocin. These elevated levels together with a low GABA level would lead to a total brain energy level that is over excited. This perfectly fits into the definition of bipolar hypomania or mania as per section F(iii-b).

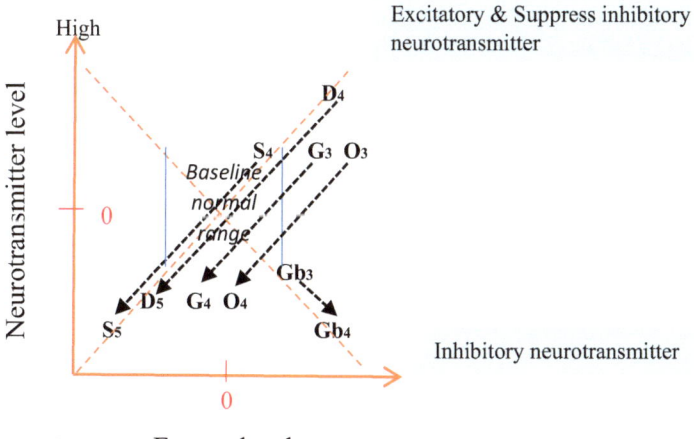

Figure F(i-2)3: Combined neurotransmitter chart – Bipolar (moderate/major depression phase)

Note:

However, an overly excited brain will attract free radical attacks [refer section F(i-1)] that can lead to all neurotransmitters being greatly depressed.

This perfectly fits into the definition of bipolar moderate-major depression as per section F(iii-b).

Note:
- Bipolar I : Consists of mania – moderate/major depression phase
- Bipolar II : Consists of hypomania – moderate/major depression phase

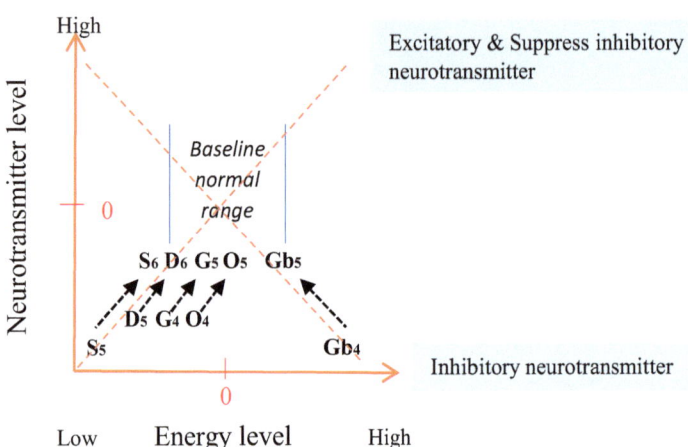

Figure F(i-2)4: Combined neurotransmitter chart – Dysthymia

Note:

With neurogenesis healing actions, the neurotransmitters are slightly elevated upwards but total brain energy level is still inhibiting and all neurotransmitters are still at a low level. This represents dysthymia (or persistent depressive disorder), a not so severe form of major depression.

(i-3) *Effective methylation, hydroxylation and oxygen level in the brain to prevent depression*

From the above, to protect against depression, an *effective methylation process [refer section C(i)], effective hydroxylation process and adequate oxygen level in the brain [refer section F figure F(i-1)2] are important in rebalancing neurotransmitter levels* to reach an equilibrium where total brain energy is within the normal range (not over excited nor over inhibited) and not amplified towards the extreme ends of the chart. Methylation is also important in detoxing neurotoxin in the brain.

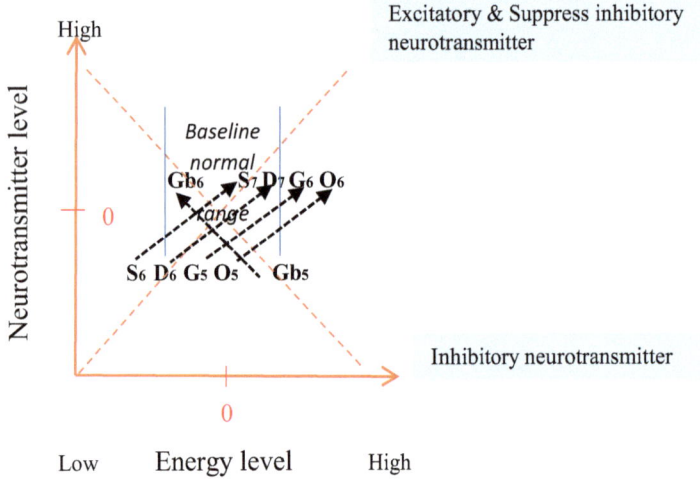

Figure F(i-3)1: Combined neurotransmitter chart – A rebalanced brain

Note:

Require effective methylation to detox neurotoxin & effective methylation, hydroxylation & adequate oxygen level in the brain to rebalance brain to baseline level.

(ii) Neurotransmitters (brain chemicals) spectrum of emotions & functions:

It is theorised here that neurotransmitter is associated with a key concept (i.e. calmness, focus, alertness, wellbeing, drivenness) and emotions are expressed when it signals to a neuron/cell via low to high variation from this base key concept.

GABA (inhibitory) - Degree of Calmness

Stimuli triggering degree of calmness, eliciting responses in physical movement and emotions (PE-positive emotions, NE- negative emotions).

Note: Stimuli is a *perception* or a *memory* of a *target subject*.

GABA level	Emotions	Movement
Very high	feeling sedated/numb/drowsy	sway like an alcoholic with very slow movements/ numb movements
High	(NE) lacking excitement (PE) very calm	slow movements
Normal	Calm	relax body
Low	(NE) anxious/ fearful/ worry/ suspicious/ mistrust (PE) excited	twitching/tics/animated movement
Very low	(NE) paranoia, dysphoria, dissociation (PE) euphoria	trembling

Figure F(ii)1: GABA level

Oxytocin (suppress inhibitory) - Degree of Focus

Focus or attention on stimuli, eliciting positive or negative emotions.

Note: Stimuli is a *perception* or a *memory* of a *target subject*.

Target subject: Other's traits which can be good or bad

Oxytocin level	Other's Good traits	Other's Bad traits
Very high	extreme focus on good traits of others (***extreme irrational joy or bliss or infatuation***)	extreme focus on bad traits of others (***extreme irrational anger/hate, blaming or projection***)
High	over focus on good traits of others (***adoration/love***)	over focus on bad traits of others (***hostility/hate/anger***)
Normal	balanced focus to good and bad traits of others (***mixture of love and agitation***)	
Low	less focus on good traits of others (***unforgiveness***)	less focus on bad traits of others (***forgiveness***)
Very low	no focus or indifference to good and bad traits of others (***total apathy towards others***) Note: Apathy- a state of indifference, a lack of interest or concern (Link 124)	

Figure F(ii)2: Oxytocin level where Target subject = Other's traits

Target subject: Self's traits which can be good or bad

Oxytocin level	Self's Good traits	Self's Bad traits
Very high	extreme focus on good traits of self (*egotistical/ aggrandization*)	extreme focus on bad traits of self [*extreme (shame, guilt, unworthiness, anger)*]
High	over focus on good traits of self (*proud, over confidence, feeling over worthy*)	over focus on bad traits of self (*shame, guilt, unworthiness, anger*)
Normal	balanced view of good and bad traits of self (*healthy confidence level*)	
Low	less focus on good traits of self (*less confidence, feeling lack of worth*)	less focus on bad traits of self (*ignorant, oblivious, unmindful, insensitive*)
Very low	no focus or indifference to good or bad traits of self (*total apathy towards sense of self-worth*)	

Figure F(ii)3: Oxytocin level where Target subject = Self's traits

Target subject: Bond strength/weakness

Note: Strong bond means entitled exclusive relationship with reciprocation of love towards each other. A weak bond is the opposite of a strong bond.

Oxytocin level	Bond strength	Bond weakness
Very high	very high focus on bond strength (*obsession*)	very high focus on bond weakness [*extremely (sad, unloved, rejected, feel betrayed, jealous)*], *vulnerability to harm/abuse/victimization*
High	high focus on bond strength [*very (happy, loved, accepted, trusting, secure)*]	high focus on bond weakness [*very (sad, unloved, rejected, feel betrayed, jealous)*]
Normal	balanced focus on bond (*happy, loved, accepted, trusting, secure but with realistic bond misgivings*)	
Low	less focus on bond strength (*uncaring, feeling distant, neglectful*)	less focus on bond weakness (*caring, closeness, attentive*)
Very low	very low focus or indifference on bond strength or weakness (*total apathy towards bond*)	

Figure F(ii)4: Oxytocin level where Target subject = Bond

Note:
- In primitive days, when a person is rejected from a secure social unit, they are vulnerable to harm from external factors.

- Oxytocin is two-faced. While it promotes feeling of love and bonding, it can cause emotional pain. *Oxytocin strengthens bad memories, triggers fear and anxiety in future stress*. Refer (Link 125) and (Link 126).

- *Too much oxytocin can result in oversensitivity to the emotions of others* (Link 127).

Glutamate (excitatory) - Degree of Alertness

Cognition alertness relates to *processing intensity* of memory, perception and learning.

Glutamate level	Memory	Perception	Learning
Very high (severe mental exhaustion)	excitoxin whereby overexcited cell leading to cell death, ***psychosis***, brain seizures		
Much higher (much higher processing intensity, mental exhaustion)	wrong memory and greater dwelling on past memories (rumination)	Delusion (fixed false interpretations)	Disturbed unorganized learnings/disturbed thoughts (i.e. jumbled up language, inappropriate thoughts)
Higher (higher processing intensity, begin to be mentally tired)	weak or gaps in memory (i.e. brain fog) and dwelling on past memories (rumination)	misperceptions or misinterpretations	weak learnings/thoughts (i.e. unable to concentrate)
High (high processing intensity)	sharp memory	perceptive	organized learnings/thoughts
Normal (normal processing intensity)	normal memory	normal perceptions	normal learnings/thoughts
Low (low processing intensity)	losing memory	losing ability to perceive adequately	losing ability to organize learnings/thoughts (i.e. unable to concentrate)
Very low (very low processing intensity) (i.e. *dementia*)	greater loss of memory	greater loss of ability to perceive adequately	greater loss of ability to organize learnings/thoughts

Figure F(ii)5: Glutamate level

Serotonin (excitatory) - Degree of Wellbeing

Feeling at ease or comfort, eliciting emotions and actions.

Serotonin level	Emotions	Actions
Very high serotonin	excessive nerve cell activity with potentially fatal ***serotonin syndrome including psychosis & cell death***	
Much higher	*Mania* (state of abnormally elevated arousal, affect and energy level)	
Higher	extremely (happy/ satisfied/ contented/comfortable)	superb sleep, superb interest in sex and food
High	very (happy/ satisfied/ contented/ comfortable)	sleep very soundly, great interest in sex and food
Normal (normal wellbeing)	happy/ satisfied/ contented/ comfortable	good sleep, interest in sex and food
Low	frustrated/ dissatisfied/ discontented/uncomfortable	mild insomnia, non interest in sex and food
Very low	very (frustrated/ dissatisfied/ discontented/uncomfortable)	insomnia, reject sex and food

Figure F(ii)6: Serotonin level

Dopamine (excitatory) - Degree of Drivenness
(Drivenness to acquire target subject, which begins with arousal, motivation, motor control/speed and reward reinforcement)

Dopamine level	Arousal	Motivation	Motor control/speed	Reward reinforcement
Very high	overexcited cells that lead to cell death, *psychosis*			
Much higher	*Mania* (state of abnormally elevated arousal, affect and energy level)			
Higher	extremely aroused (*extremely interested/ lustful*)	extremely motivated [*extremely (purposeful/ determined/ motivated/ looking forward/ hopeful*)]	extremely high speed of action (*very impulsive & disinhibited*)	extremely reward reinforcement oriented (*wanting acknowledgement/wanting to be appreciated*) (If acquired- *extremely pleasurable or addictive, euphoria, extremely grateful, feeling extremely capable*) (if not acquired- *extremely displeased/ extremely unhappy or sad/ extremely frustrated/ extremely overwhelmed/ extremely envious*)
High	high arousal (*highly interested*)	high motivation [*very (purposeful/ determined/ motivated/ looking forward/hopeful*)]	high speed of action (*impulsive and disinhibited*)	high reward reinforcement (If acquired-*highly pleasurable or addictive, very happy, very grateful, feeling very capable*) (If not acquired-*highly displeased/ very unhappy or sad/ very frustrated/ very overwhelmed/ very envious*)
Normal	measured level of arousal (*interested*)	measured level of motivation (*purposeful/ determined/ motivated/ looking forward/hopeful*)	measured speed of action (*normal reaction*)	measured level of reward reinforcement (if acquired- *pleasurable/ happy/ grateful/ feeling able to cope*)(if not acquired-*not so pleased/ unhappy or sad/ frustrated/ overwhelmed/ envious*)
Low	low arousal (*lacking interest*)	low motivation [*feeling losing (a sense of purpose/ direction/ motivation/ meaning in life/hope)*]	low speed of action (*slow reaction*)	low reward reinforcement (*slight indifference whether there is reward for efforts- moderate apathy*)
Very low	very low arousal (*very lacking in interest*)	very low motivation [*very lacking in (a sense of purpose/ direction/ motivation/ meaning in life/hope)*]	very low speed of action (*very slow reaction*)	very low reward reinforcement (*indifference whether there is reward for efforts-total apathy*)

Figure F(ii)7: Dopamine level

(iii) Why Depression and Mania happens

iii-a) It is theorized here that *depression happens when total brain energy is negative or inhibiting* (feeling of oppressiveness, rather than feeling alive). There are various subtypes of depression:
- sad based depression
- fear based depression
- angry based depression
- biological based depression
- tired based depression
- borderline depression or now termed as Borderline Personality Disorder (it is actually a hybrid form of depression, fluctuating between normalcy and extreme emotions)
- dysthymia
- bipolar depression
- major depression with anxiety

iii-b) *If total brain energy level is excitatory and either serotonin or dopamine level is at a much higher to very high level, then hypomania or mania occurs.* However, an overly excited brain will attract free radical attacks [refer section F(i-1)] that can lead to all neurotransmitters being depressed. Hence, a total brain energy level that is over excited can turn into a total brain energy level that is overly inhibiting. This is a feature of Bipolar where mood fluctuates between hypomania/mania - moderate depression/major depression.

iii-c) The examples below will require reference to the neurotransmitter type & levels (i.e. whether which neurotransmitter is involved and whether the level is high or low) in section F(ii) above. The quantum used is just for explanatory purposes and the assumption that the stress situation depicted is prolonged (chronic). "+" represents the extreme upper end level while "-" represents the extreme lower end level of the neurotransmitter.

Example of sad based depression
Target subject: Relationship loss

When we lose a relationship, we feel hopeless [low dopamine (-1)] and frustrated [low serotonin (-1)]. We blame ourselves for the loss and this will lower our self-worth [low oxytocin (-1)]. When we continuously dwell and mourn for the relationship loss [high glutamate (+2)] & [high oxytocin (+2)], we miss the person even more and feel even more hopeless [lower dopamine (-2)] and more frustrated [lower serotonin (-2)]. We worry we will not find a future relationship [low GABA (-1)].

	Workings	Over exciting	Inhibiting	**Net total**
GABA	-(-1)	+1		
Glutamate	+2	+2		
Serotonin	(-1-2)		-3	
Dopamine	(-1-2)		-3	
Oxytocin	(-1+2)	+1		
Brain energy		+4	-6	**-2**

Figure F(iii)1: Sad based depression case study

Note: In general, a sad based depression is characterized by a neurotransmitter profile where there are low levels of serotonin, dopamine, GABA and high levels of oxytocin, glutamate.

Example of a fear based depression
Target subject: Robber

When we fear a robber is about to harm us [low GABA (-1)] and our wellbeing is jeopardized [low serotonin (-3)], we need to be mentally alert [high glutamate (+2)] and focus on how to acquire safety from the robber [high oxytocin (+2)], [high dopamine (+3)]. Preliminary accumulative brain energy is overly excited, leading to free radical attacks which depress all neurotransmitters by (-1), in particular serotonin (-3) and dopamine (-2).

	Workings	Preliminary total with overly excited brain	Free radical attacks depress all neurotransmitters, in particular serotonin & dopamine	Net total
GABA	-(-1)	+1	-(-1)	-(-2)
Glutamate	+2	+2	-1	+1
Serotonin	-3	-3	-3	-6
Dopamine	+3	+3	-2	+1
Oxytocin	+2	+2	-1	+1
Brain energy		**+5**	**-6**	**-1**

Figure F(iii)2: Fear based depression case study

Note: In general, a fear based depression is characterized by a neurotransmitter profile where there are low levels of serotonin, GABA and high levels of glutamate, oxytocin, dopamine.

Example of a major depression with anxiety
Target subject: Unfaithful spouse

An unfaithful spouse will lead to severe emotional stress where we will feel extremely frustrated [low serotonin (-3)], angry [high oxytocin (+2)], low self-worth [low oxytocin (-1)], anxious [low GABA (-2)], very unhappy or sad [high dopamine (+2)] and intensely think of ways to deal with the challenging situation [high glutamate (+1)]. Preliminary accumulative brain energy is overly excited, leading to free radical attacks which depress all neurotransmitters by (-2), in particular serotonin (-3) and dopamine (-3).

	Workings	Preliminary total with overly excited brain	Free radical attacks depress all neurotransmitters, in particular serotonin & dopamine	Net total
GABA	-(-2)	+2	-(-2)	-(-4)
Glutamate	+1	+1	-2	-1
Serotonin	-3	-3	-3	-6
Dopamine	+2	+2	-3	-1
Oxytocin	+2-1	+1	-2	-1
Brain energy		**+3**	**-8**	**-5**

Figure F(iii)3: Major depression with anxiety case study

Note: In general, a major depression with anxiety is characterized by a neurotransmitter profile where there are low levels of GABA, glutamate, dopamine, oxytocin and very low level for serotonin.

Example of an angry based depression
Target subject: Retrenchment

When we lose our job, we feel lost [low dopamine (-2)] and rejected by the company [high oxytocin (+1)]. We start to worry for our stream of income [low GABA (-1)] and not in the mood to eat [low serotonin (-2)] but think of ways in finding the next job [high glutamate (+1)].

	Workings	Over exciting	Inhibiting	Net total
GABA	-(-1)	+1		
Glutamate	+1	+1		
Serotonin	-2		-2	
Dopamine	-2		-2	
Oxytocin	+1	+1		
Brain energy		+3	-4	**-1**

Figure F(iii)4: Angry based depression case study

Note: In general, an angry based depression is characterized by a neurotransmitter profile where there are low levels of serotonin, dopamine, GABA and high levels of glutamate, oxytocin.

Example of a biological based depression
Target subject: Bad diet

Due to a low intake of good probiotic, the gut has more bad bacteria, which leads to more toxin build up and cause one to easily fall sick [low serotonin (-1)].

	Workings	Over exciting	Inhibiting	Net total
GABA				
Glutamate				
Serotonin	-1		-1	
Dopamine				
Oxytocin				
Brain energy			-1	**-1**

Figure F(iii)6: Biological based depression case study

Note: In general, a biological based depression is characterized by a neurotransmitter profile where there is a low level of serotonin while GABA, glutamate, dopamine and oxytocin are in the normal range.

Example of a tired based depression
Target subject: Overworked body (i.e. Excessive workload)

When we overworked our body running through the list of to-do [high glutamate (+1)], [high dopamine (+1)], we may be too busy and start to miss meals [insufficient calorie intake leading to exhaustion and trembling, thus, low GABA (-1)]. We feel extremely tired [low serotonin (-5)] and become irritable at others [high oxytocin (+1)].

	Workings	Over exciting	Inhibiting	**Net total**
GABA	-(-1)	+1		
Glutamate	+1	+1		
Serotonin	-5		-5	
Dopamine	+1	+1		
Oxytocin	+1	+1		
Brain energy		+4	-5	**-1**

Figure F(iii)7: Tired based depression case study

Note: In general, a tired based depression is characterized by a neurotransmitter profile where there are low levels of serotonin, GABA and high levels of glutamate, oxytocin, dopamine.

iii-d) Therefore, low levels of only serotonin or dopamine do not necessarily mean there will be depression. We need to calculate the entire brain energy level. Low serotonin and dopamine levels measured via urine analysis will most likely indicate the body is lacking in some protein (i.e. tryptophan and tyrosine), which are ingredients to make serotonin and dopamine respectively. (Note: there is a controversy whether measurement via urine represents levels in the brain due to the blood brain barrier, but it may give an approximation).

(G) Case study: Major depression with anxiety, BPD/Borderline depression, Bipolar and Dysthymia

Stage 1: Grief
When a man loses a relationship, he feels hopeless [low dopamine (-1)], sad [high oxytocin (+1)], anxious [low GABA (-1)] and frustrated [low serotonin (-1)] as he thinks about the ex [high glutamate (+1)]. He blames himself for the loss and this will lower his self-worth [low oxytocin (-1)].

Stage 2: Anxiety
When he moves past the grief stage of the loss, and as time passes on, he dwells over the loss [higher oxytocin (+2)], [higher glutamate (+1)] and becomes more anxious [lower GABA (-1)] on the worry whether will he be able to meet the right person [higher dopamine (+2)] in the future. If he has yet to encounter the person, he becomes very frustrated [lower serotonin (-2)].

Note: Excessive glutamate is a neurotoxin which damages the brain and too high dopamine and oxytocin signalling attract free radicals that damage the brain (oxidative stress). In particular, estrogen receptor beta (ERβ) at oxytocin-containing cells, glutamate, dopamine and oxytocin receptors of the brain [refer section F(i-1)]. Damages at the brain result in malabsorption of water, oxygen and nutrients. A depressed brain oxygen level will further depress all neurotransmitter levels by (-3) but greatly depresses serotonin (-6) and dopamine (-3). *This is when major depression with anxiety occurs*.

Stage 3: Medication for depression
Upon Lexapro antidepressant intake, it will increase all neurotransmitter levels [serotonin (+3), dopamine (+3) while the rest (+2)] as antidepressants are believed to have antioxidant properties [refer section F(i-1)]. However, the antidepressant intake was stopped once the major depression ceases, not knowing that the brain is still weak and not properly rejuvenated. *A weak brain due to methylation issues will not be able to readjust all the neurotransmitters back to normal baseline level* (Link 128). Hence, the major depression with anxiety now turns into a form of resistant depression, termed as *Borderline depression*, with features of amplification of oxytocin, dopamine, glutamate to borderline high levels while serotonin and GABA are amplified toward borderline low levels and the total brain energy is in equilibrium. The BPD or Borderline depression symptoms manifest during the scenarios below.

Stage 4: Normal life worries & frustrations
Daily life stressors can cause him worries [lower GABA (-2)] and frustrations [lower serotonin (-2)] and thus more headaches [higher glutamate (+2)] as he tries to resolve the problems [higher dopamine (+2)]. He may unload his frustrations to others (blaming/projection) as a way to cope with his emotional pain [high oxytocin (+2)]. Accumulatively, normal life worries and frustrations create more total excitatory energy for the brain. This will lead to more free radical attacks at the brain causing a depressed oxygen brain environment which further depress all neurotransmitter levels by (-1) but greatly depresses serotonin (-4) and dopamine (-2).

	Stage 1: Sadness/Grief	Accumulative	Stage 2: Anxiety & free radical attacks	Accumulative	Stage 3: Antidepressant intake for someone with MTHFR or methylation defects	Accumulative (without efficient methylation, hence, neurotransmitters not brought back to baseline)	Stage 4: Normal life worries & frustrations	Accumulative
GABA	-1	-(-1)	-(-1-3)	-(-5)	+2	-(-3)	-(-2) and -(-1)	-(-6)
Glutamate	+1	+1	+1-3	-1	+2	+1	+2-1	+2
Dopamine	-1	-1	+2-3	-2	+3	+1	+2-2	+1
Oxytocin	+1, -1	0	+2-3	-1	+2	+1	+2-1	+2
Serotonin	-1	-1	-2-6	-9	+3	-6	-2-4	-12
Over excited brain energy		+2		+5		+6		+11
Inhibiting brain energy		-2		-13		-6		-12
Total brain energy		0, no depression		-8 (Major depression with anxiety disorder where all neurotransmitters are low, especially serotonin)		0 (no major depression but serotonin & GABA still borderline low while glutamate, oxytocin, dopamine are borderline high, a feature of BPD/ Borderline)		-1, Borderline depression

Figure G1: Demonstration of how Major depression with anxiety and BPD/Borderline depression occur

Based on the above chart, this male is still depressed after the Lexapro antidepressant medication. But, the depression has transformed from Major depression with anxiety disorder into Borderline depression and the borderline behaviour is normally exhibited when he is anxious/ frustrated or when there are increases in estrogen level primarily due to greater aromatization of testosterone to estradiol as a result of MetS factors (i.e. inflammation, insulin resistance, obesity). *Borderline depression is characterised by very high glutamate, oxytocin, dopamine levels and very low GABA and serotonin levels.* He needs to rebalance via effective methylation, effective hydroxylation and adequate oxygen level in the brain [refer section F(i-3)] to bring all neurotransmitter levels back to baseline normal levels.

Refer (Link 129), (Link 130) and (Link 131)

Stage 5: Bipolar I mania phase
A borderline depression level combined with further excessive protein intake (i.e. tryptophan and tyrosine which are dietary precursors to serotonin and dopamine respectively), can further elevate serotonin (+6) and dopamine (+6) to higher levels. As such, dopamine would be at an extremely high level alongside high levels of glutamate and oxytocin. These elevated levels together with a low GABA level would lead to an overly excited brain energy level. This perfectly fits into the definition of hypomania or mania as per section F(iii-b).

Stage 6: Bipolar I major depression phase
However, an overly excited brain will attract free radical attacks [refer section F(i-1)] that can lead to all neurotransmitters being greatly depressed by (-4) and in particular serotonin and dopamine by (-10). This perfectly fits into the definition of major depression as per section F(iii-b).

Stage 7: Dysthymia phase
Practising natural healing, he undertakes neurogenesis actions (i.e. meditation, deep breathing exercises) which calm his anxieties, thus elevating GABA (+6). Additionally, he indulges in fulfilling activities (i.e. travels) that increase his feeling of wellbeing, thus elevating serotonin (+8). He also meets up with friends and these interactions will increase his friendship bonds (oxytocin, +2), increase his knowledge through chats/sharings (glutamate, +2) and increase his pleasure (dopamine, +2).

Radical theory on MetS & Depression

	From Figure G1: Accumulative (without efficient methylation, hence, neurotransmitters not brought back to baseline)	Stage 5: Excessive protein intake elevates serotonin and dopamine	Accumulative	Stage 6: Free radical attacks an over excited brain, depressing all neurotransmitters	Accumulative	Stage 7: Neurogenesis healing actions	Accumulative
GABA	-(-3)		-(-3)	-(-4)	-(-7)	+6	-(-1)
Glutamate	+1		+1	-4	-3	+2	-1
Dopamine	+1	+6	+7	-10	-3	+2	-1
Oxytocin	+1		+1	-4	-3	+2	-1
Serotonin	-6	+6	0	-10	-10	+8	-2
Over excited brain energy	+6		+12		+7		+1
Inhibiting brain energy	-6				-19		-5
Total brain energy	0 (no major depression but serotonin & GABA still borderline low while glutamate, oxytocin, dopamine are borderline high, a feature of BPD/ Borderline)		+12 (Bipolar I mania where there are high levels of oxytocin & glutamate, very high dopamine, normal baseline level for serotonin while GABA is at a low level)		-12 (Bipolar I major depression with anxiety disorder where all neurotransmitters are low, especially serotonin)		-4 (Dysthymia where all neurotransmitters are low but total inhibiting brain energy is lesser than major depression)

Figure G3: Demonstration of how Bipolar mania-major depression and as well as Dysthymia occur

From figure G1 and G3, the mood disorders are plotted along the mania – depression spectrum along with their calculated total brain energy level.

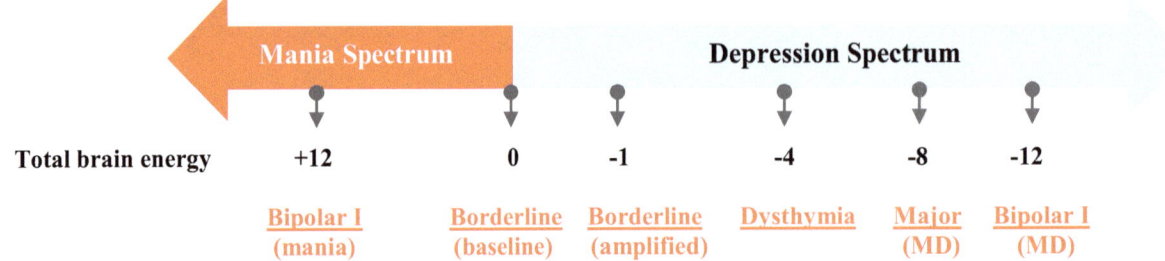

Note: MD denotes Major depression

(H) Summary of depression neurotransmitter profiles

Depression type	GABA	Glutamate	Serotonin	Dopamine	Oxytocin
Sad	Low	High	Low	Low	High
Fear	Low	High	Low	High	High
Angry	Low	High	Low	Low	High
Biological	Normal	Normal	Low	Normal	Normal
Tired	Low	High	Low	High	High
Borderline	Low	High	Low	High	High
Dysthymia	Low	Low	Low	Low	Low
Bipolar (hypomania-mania)	Low	High	Baseline	Very high	High
Bipolar (moderate depression-major depression)	Low	Low	Low or very low	Low	Low
Major depression with anxiety	Low	Low	Very low	Low	Low

Figure H1: Depression neurotransmitter profiles

Note:
Refer to section E under the column "affected organs = brain" to find out the ways to determine the neurotransmitter profile.

(I) Neurotransmitter imbalance and ways to rebalance

Neurotransmitter imbalance root causes	Ways to rebalance

GABA level is low:
1. Insufficient glucose diet intake [refer section C(ii-4)] leads to anxiety.
2. Habit of worrying creates anxiety.
 	
3. Activation estrogen receptor alpha > estrogen receptor beta [refer section A(ii)].
4. Depressed oxygen level in the brain leads to low GABA level [refer section F(i-1)].
	1. Higher intake of complex carbohydrate.
	2. a) Undertake mindfulness techniques, deep breathing & yoga.
	   b) Undertake epsom bath (magnesium) with essential oils (lemon balm, passionflower).
	   c) Calm anxieties via tea consumption (as it consists theanine, an amino acid which boosts GABA level).
	3. Intake of protein & good oil to regenerate damaged receptor and antioxidant to counter oxidative stress.
	4. Higher antioxidant (i.e. Vitamin C & E, green tea, blueberry, turmeric) intake to counter oxidative stress, protein & good oil to regenerate brain cells.
	5. Refer an excellent article on how to increase GABA (Link 132).

Glutamate level is high:
1. Intense mental activity or dwelling/ruminating on a subject leads to high glutamate.
2. Thereafter, excessive glutamate causes excitoxicity. Combined with the influx of calcium to the over excited cell, will destroy nerve cell.
 	
(refer Link 133)
	1. Avoid dwelling/ruminating on a subject.
	2. a) Intake of antioxidant to counter oxidative stress.
	   b) Vitamin D (i.e. sun exposure) and K (i.e. dark leafy greens) intake to re-establish calcium balance.
	   c) Increase magnesium to balance calcium.
	   d) Zinc intake to limit glutamate damage.
	   e) Reduce gluten and casein (found in cow's milk) intake to control glutamate level.
	   f) Avoid glutamine supplements and MSG food that can increase glutamate.

Glutamate level is low: 1. Lack of mental usage which worsens mental capacity. 2. Protein catabolisation in times of chronic stress that depletes glutamine, and therefore glutamate level in the body [refer section C(ii-1)]. 3. Low intake of protein (i.e. glutamine which is a precursor to glutamate). 4. Depressed oxygen level in the brain leads to low glutamate level [refer section F(i-1)].	1. Practise mental exercises to increase glutamate. 2. Practise stress management. 3. Increase protein or glutamine supplements intake to increase glutamate. 4. Higher antioxidant (i.e. Vitamin C & E, green tea, blueberry, turmeric) intake to counter oxidative stress, protein & good oil to regenerate brain cells.

Neurotransmitter imbalance root causes	Ways to rebalance
Serotonin level is low:	
1. Elevated MAO-A activity due to stress which decreases serotonin availability [refer section F(i-2)].	1. a) Intake of precursor for serotonin such as vitamin B6, 5-HTP (a type of protein). b) Practise stress management.
2. Activation estrogen receptor alpha > estrogen receptor beta [refer section A(ii)].	2. Intake of protein and good oil to regenerate damaged receptor and antioxidant to counter oxidative stress.
3. Lack of protein intake (i.e. tryptophan, a precursor to serotonin).	3. Increase protein consumption.
4. Depressed oxygen level in the brain leading to reduced tryptophan hydrolase and consequently very low serotonin level [refer section F(i-1)].	4. Higher antioxidant (i.e. Vitamin C & E, green tea, blueberry, turmeric) intake to counter oxidative stress, protein & good oil to regenerate brain cells.
Dopamine level is high:	
1. Intense mental activity or dwelling/ruminating on a subject leads to high dopamine.	1. Avoid dwelling/ruminating on a subject.
2. Decrease in COMT activity due to stress, which increases dopamine in the brain [refer section F(i-2)].	2. a) Supplement with magnesium, vitamin C and Bs. b) Practise stress management.
3. Excessive protein elevates tyrosine, a precursor to dopamine.	3. Reduce protein intake.
Dopamine level is low:	
1. Depressed oxygen level in the brain leading to reduced tyrosine hydrolase and consequently very low dopamine level [refer section F(i-1)].	1. Higher antioxidant (i.e. Vitamin C & E, green tea, blueberry, turmeric) intake to counter oxidative stress, protein & good oil to regenerate brain cells.
2. Lack of protein intake (i.e. tyrosine, a precursor to dopamine).	2. Increase protein consumption.
Oxytocin level is high:	
1. Intense mental activity or dwelling/ruminating on a subject leads to high oxytocin.	1. Avoid dwelling/ruminating on a subject.
2. Anxiety (low GABA) triggers 5 alpha reductase that amplifies oxytocin [refer section A(ii)].	2. Undertake mindfulness techniques.
3. The triggering of 5 alpha reductase can lead to oxidative stress and inflammation for the brain.	3. Intake of 2-3 months of fish oil (antioxidant & anti-inflammatory oil) with dosage of 1000mg and above of EPA & DHA shows promising treatment for depression (i.e. BPD) [Link 134]. Intake of vitamin D, carminitine herbs (i.e. garlic, onion), anti-inflammatory diet to counter inflammation.
4. Anxiety problems could be caused by insufficient glucose diet intake [refer section C(ii-4)].	4. Increase complex carb intake.
Oxytocin level is low:	
1. Depressed oxygen level in the brain leads to low oxytocin level [refer section F(i-1)].	1. Higher antioxidant (i.e. Vitamin C & E, green tea, blueberry, turmeric) intake to counter oxidative stress, protein & good oil to regenerate brain cells.

Figure I1: Neurotransmitter imbalance and ways to rebalance

Summary of nutrients, supplementation and healing actions based on figure I1 above:

Overall neurotransmitter imbalance	Summary nutrients, supplementation & healing actions to rebalance
1. Methylation problems which cause non rebalance of all neurotransmitters back to baseline levels [refer section F(i-3) and C(i)].	1. Intake of multivitamin & mineral with higher vitamins (all active vitamin Bs including B8-inositol, B9-folate, B12-methylcobalamin), C and minerals zinc & magnesium to rebalance methylation.
2. Mental stress creates free radical attacks to the brain, leading to a state of depressed oxygen level in the brain, weakening the brain [refer section F(i-1)].	2. a) Intake of antioxidant i.e. green tea, blueberries, turmeric, fish oil, vitamin C and E to counter oxidative stress. b) Intake of vitamin D, carminitine herbs (i.e. garlic, onion), anti-inflammatory diet to counter inflammation. c) Increase complex carbohydrate to reduce anxieties. d) Intake of good oil (i.e. flax seed/fish oil) to repair cell membrane. e) Intake of complete liquid protein (i.e. soya, almond milk) to repair cell: • Soya, a protein and phytoestrogen, mimics estrogen in protection against oxidative stress in the liver and brain mitochondria without the feminising and tumour promotion properties (Link 135). • Phytoestrogens, especially isoflavones, have an affinity with estrogen receptor beta (ERβ) rather than estrogen receptor alpha (ERα) (Link 136). *Caution*: For those with high neuronal activity (i.e. high dopamine/ serotonin/ glutamate) manifested as hypomania/ mania/ racing thoughts or rapid speech, the intake of protein should be reduced in the beginning while other steps above are undertaken and thereafter, to gradually increase protein consumption to repair cell. 3. Stress relieving management & practices (i.e. mindfulness, deep breathing, yoga, epsom bath with magnesium, tea consumption). 4. Avoid dwelling/rumination.

Figure I2: Overall neurotransmitter imbalance and summary ways to rebalance

Note 1:
To consult a naturopathic doctor on the suitability of the supplements/herbs, according to your body chemistry.

Note 2: **Mindfulness-based intervention lowers anxiety**

It should be noted that mindfulness interventions appear to bring about an improvement in symptoms characteristic of Borderline depression/BPD and some who underwent mindfulness-based treatment no longer meet the diagnostic criteria for BPD (this correlates with Dialectical Behaviour Therapy (DBT) as mindfulness is central to all skills in DBT), refer (Link 137).

(J) Inconsistent findings on testosterone therapy in relieving depression

- Testosterone therapy will likely improve anxiety level in men, (Link 138).

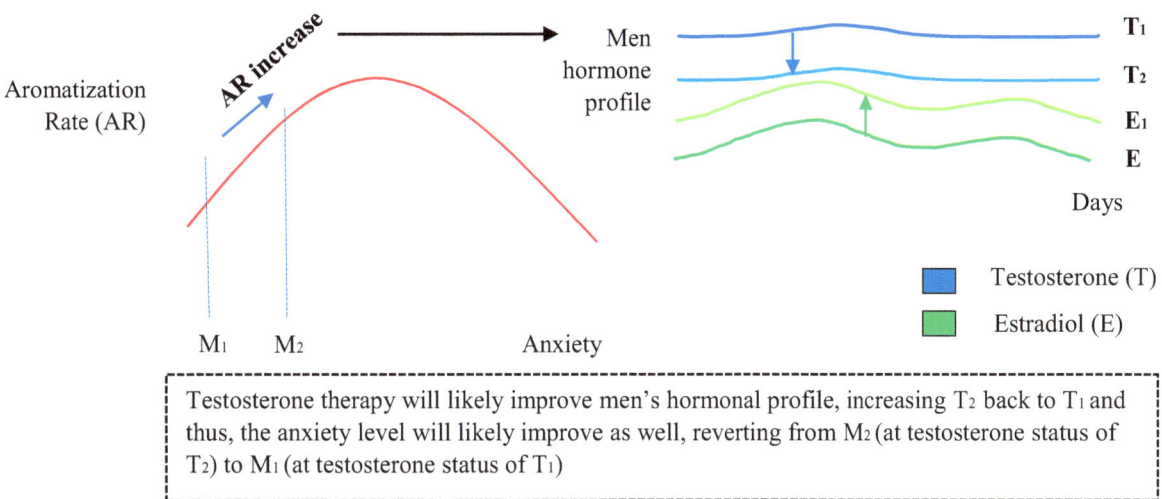

Figure J1: Theoretically, testosterone therapy will improve anxiety level in men

- Nonetheless, due to discrepancies between studies, testosterone treatment for men with depression is not recommended, although there is a strong possibility that it might benefit some men. [Refer (Link 139) and (Link 140)].
- In the author's opinion, this could be due to the fact that testosterone (T) can be transformed either (with reference to figure A5):
  - to DHT via 5 alpha reductase enzyme (triggered by anxiety), which then activates estrogen receptor beta (ERβ) in the brain, leading to further activation of oxytocin/dopamine and glutamate in the brain, thus increasing the brain's excitatory energy level. Hence, if the original state of the brain already has damaged oxytocin/dopamine and glutamate receptors, further excitement may induce more damage to these receptors
  - to estradiol (E) via aromatase enzyme (where the aromatization rate is influenced by MetS factors such as inflammation, insulin resistance and obesity). If the aromatization rate increases due to MetS factors, hence, testosterone increasingly will be transformed to estradiol (i.e. worsening T/E ratio), leading to the feminization of men. This may cause the men to feel discontentment over his physical appearance, thus, lowering serotonin level
  - Hence, the above items may lead to further depression rather than the reversal of depression

Note :
Do consult with a qualified doctor with regards to any hormone therapy, as there is a need to establish any gap in hormone levels (based on factors such as age, gender etc.) prior to any application of hormonal treatment.

- Additionally, though testosterone therapy will likely improve men's anxiety level, nonetheless, anxiety (or low GABA level) is just one component within the depression neurotransmitter profile:

ERβ damage due to overexertion of the brain triggered by anxiety (low GABA)	Depression type	GABA	Glutamate	Serotonin	Dopamine	Oxytocin
Low	Borderline	Low	High	Low	High	High
Moderate	Dysthymia	Low	Low	Low	Low	Low
High	Bipolar (hypomania-mania)	Low	High	Baseline	Very high	High
	Bipolar (moderate depression-major depression)	Low	Low	Low or very low	Low	Low
Extreme	Major depression with anxiety	Low	Low	Very low	Low	Low

Figure J2: Depression neurotransmitter profile and its association with anxiety level (i.e. low GABA)

- Testosterone therapy will reduce anxiety and excitability of the brain's total energy (i.e. an increase in GABA level and generally, a decrease in oxytocin/dopamine/glutamate level)
- Hence, testosterone therapy will likely improve depression types where these is over excitement of the brain, such as Borderline depression and Bipolar (hypomania-mania)

(K) *Common concise protocol & nutrient intake to rectify MetS and Depression (BPD/Borderline depression, Dysthymia, Bipolar and Major depression with anxiety)*

Protocol
1-Restore strength of neuroendocrine organs that require specialize treatment: liver, gut and adrenal. The other remaining neuroendocrine organs (refer section E) will be restored when protocol 2 is undertaken.
2-Replenish nutrients to its optimal level.

Protocol 1: Restoring organs' strength

Organs	Examples	Rationale	Supplements			
			Seeking Health multivitamin (Optimal Plus line if concurrent approach) (4 pills)	Any brand of fish oil	Go Healthy Go Probiotic 75 billion (1 pill)	Any brand of complete protein powder
Liver	Milk thistle	Improve detoxification & digestion	Optimal Plus line- Milk thistle*	Fish oil (dosage: at least 1000mg)		
Gut	Probiotics Protein powder	Improve good bacteria. Heal leaky gut			Probiotics	Complete protein
Adrenal	Ashwagandha, Rhodiola rosea	Rebalance stress response	Optimal Plus line- Ashwagandha**			

Note *: Can opt for a single supplement to rejuvenate the liver in replacement of Seeking Health Optimal Plus multivitamin. Recommended supplement: 1 bottle of A. Vogel Liver Gallbladder drops.

Note **: Can opt for a single supplement to rejuvenate the adrenal in replacement of Seeking Health Optimal Plus multivitamin. Recommended supplement: 1 bottle of Rhodiola rosea 250mg.

Protocol 2: Replenishing nutrients

Nutrient	Examples	Rationale	Supplements		
			Seeking Health multivitamin (Optimal line if phased approach) (4 pills)	Any brand of fish oil	Any brand of complete protein powder
Protein	Higher liquid protein (i.e. soy, almond milk, bone broth)	To heal cells damaged by free radicals and counter effects of protein catabolisation. Improve hydroxylation			Complete protein
Essential fatty acid	Higher essential fatty acid (i.e. more than 1000mg fish oil or flax seed oil)	To heal membrane cells damaged by free radicals as membrane consists of essential fatty acid. To reduce 5 alpha reductase and inflammation. Improve hydroxylation		Fish oil (dosage: at least 1000mg)	

Nutrient	Examples	Rationale	Supplements		
			Seeking Health multivitamin (Optimal line if phased approach) (4 pills)	Any brand of fish oil	Any brand of complete protein powder
Antioxidant	Higher antioxidant (i.e. blueberries, fish oil (1000mg), flax seed oil, green tea, turmeric, vitamin C, E)	To counter oxidative stress stemming from free radical damages	Vitamin C, E, turmeric and other antioxidant ingredients	Fish oil (dosage: at least 1000mg)	
Vitamins & Minerals	Higher vitamins (must have all active Bs including B8-inositol, B9-folate, B12-methylcobalamin, C,A,D,E,K) and mineral zinc, magnesium	Crucial for body processes (i.e. methylation, growth/healing & immunity)	Higher vitamins (must have all active Bs including B8-inositol, B9-folate, B12-methylcobalamin, C,A,D,E,K) and mineral zinc, magnesium		
Complex carbo-hydrate	Oats	Adequate energy level. Too much simple carb may lead to obesity, insulin resistance & diabetes while too little carb creates anxiety			
Fibre	Fruits & vegetables	Improve methylation, cholesterol	Fruits & vegetables blend		
Water	Sufficient water	Crucial for hydroxylation			

Figure K1: Common protocol & nutrient intake to rectify MetS, BPD/Borderline depression, Dysthymia, Bipolar and Major depression with anxiety

Note 1: The above concise healing protocols are a summarization based on Section E and Section I.

Note 2: Protocol timing options and supplement brand
- **Phased approach (healing in 2 steps 6 supplements)** : undertake protocol 1 first to focus on restoring the organs' strength via the following supplements:
    o A. Vogel's Liver Gallbladder drops, formulated by a known naturopath (1 bottle) [Link 141],
    o Go Healthy Go Probiotic which contains the right type of probiotic strains [Link 142] beneficial for mental & physical health (1 bottle) [Link 143],
    o any brand of rhodiola rosea 250mg (1 bottle),
    o any brand of fish oil (1 bottle) and
    o any brand of complete protein powder (1 bottle).

Thereafter, to replenish nutrients level as per protocol 2 via the supplements from:

   o Seeking Health Optimal multivitamin line, formulated by a naturopathic doctor and MTHFR expert [Link 144], continue with the fish oil & complete protein powder.

Longer duration to complete protocol 1 & 2 but will help to build a strong foundation.

- **Concurrent approach (healing in 1 step 4 supplements)**: undertake protocol 1 & 2 concurrently via supplements from Seeking Health *Optimal Plus* multivitamin line (1 bottle), Go Healthy Go Probiotic (1 bottle), any brand of fish oil (1 bottle) and any brand of complete protein powder (1 bottle). Shorter duration to complete protocol 1 & 2.
- If your body is tested via the inflammation test (refer section E) to be highly inflammatory, apart from the fish oil, an addition of flax seed oil can further boost up the anti-inflammatory actions and reduce 5 alpha reductase.
- It should be noted that 2-3 months of fish oil (1000mg and above of EPA & DHA) shows promising treatment for BPD.
- *Caution*: For those with high neuronal activity (i.e. high dopamine/ serotonin/ glutamate) manifested as hypomania/ mania/ racing thoughts or rapid speech, the intake of protein (i.e. protein or glutamine powder) should be reduced in the beginning while other steps mentioned above are undertaken and thereafter, to gradually increase protein consumption to repair cell.
- To consult a naturopathic doctor for your suitability of the supplements above.

Note 3: Adequate nutrition: Food, supplements, exercise and detoxification diary

Establishing a food diary for a minimum of 2 months (to instil a lifestyle change discipline) will help to track and ensure the proper intake of food (50% vegetable/fruits/nuts with a focus on antioxidant food, 25% quality protein e.g. fish, 25% complex carb, essential fatty acid, 8 glasses water) & the supplements above to replenish nutrients to its adequate level. To also track for exercise type & duration (moderate exercise for 30 minutes a day) as well as number of poop (detoxification) undertaken per day. Example:

Day	Breakfast	Lunch	Dinner	Hydration	Supplements	Exercise	Poop
1	Almond milk with oats, blueberries*, nuts, flaxseed oil* Vegetable juice	Salad with olive oil* Roast chicken with quinoa Apple	Stir fry vegetable with olive oil* Steam turmeric* fish* with brown rice Pear	7 glasses of water 1 cup of green tea*	Multivitamin, mineral, fibre & antioxidants Fish oil Probiotic Protein powder	30 minutes of moderate exercises	Once

Figure K2: Example of a "Food, supplements, exercise and detoxification" diary

- Consultation with a dietician/ nutritionist or a self-help nutrition book will help to increase one's nutritional knowledge. Do note that there are bad and good carbohydrate/oils/protein. For example, simple carbohydrate (i.e. white rice) is easily converted to sugar which leads to an increase in the body's free radicals and inflammation. Vegetable oils (which are chemically processed) are not as good compared to olive and flax seed oil (pressed oils). Fish (protein) grown in mercury tainted seas are toxic.

- Note:
  Items denoted with " * " are antioxidant food (i.e. blueberries, flax seed oil, fish oil from fish, olive oil, turmeric, green tea).

Note 4: Adequate mental coping: Regulate emotions and de-stressing techniques
- Daily journaling of emotions and self-soothing techniques to regulate back emotions (i.e. either manual or usage of an artificial intelligence mobile application called "Youper") or seek help from a qualified BPD/depression/anxiety psychologist.
- Record daily de-stressing techniques applied (i.e. meditation, deep breathing).

(L) Implications for physical and mental health

Physical health:
- A modern concise quick approach to protect health in times of stress is to take higher levels of protein shake with a multivitamin & mineral especially formulated with antioxidants, higher levels of vitamin Bs in active forms, C,A,D,E,K and minerals zinc & magnesium. To combine with good fats i.e. flax seed oil and fish oil. This is to ensure replenishment of amino acids, vitamins, minerals, antioxidant and good fats.

- Occasional fasting with just water and a rainbow colour of vegetables/fruits/nuts (containing antioxidant, vitamin & mineral, fats, fibre properties) whilst reducing free radical production stemming from carbohydrate digestion processes will do wonders for our health.

- Cholesterol profile testing and observation of severe acne on the face are the fastest way to detect the source of stress on our overall health. For example, acne on the forehead denotes over emotional mental stress with overworking of the brain whilst acne on the lower chin area denotes anxious stress and overworking of the liver in stress handling [refer D(i-5)]. Meanwhile, high total cholesterol implies our fertility is suppressed, high LDL cholesterol implies our body is androgenic and low HDL cholesterol implies our digestion is weak [refer D(iii)]. High triglycerides denote metabolic issues [refer D(i-1)].

Mental health:
- Words have energy (excitatory or inhibitory). We can literally think ourselves into depression or cause others to go into depression through our words.

- Our habitual ways of thinking (positive: forgiveness & love vs. negative: unforgiveness, bitterness, hate & worry) can either promote or decrease our mental health. Thus, mindfulness and dwelling on positive thoughts can prevent depression.

- It is anticipated that each mental health condition (i.e. bipolar, major depression, etc.) will have its own neurotransmitter profile.

- During antidepressant intakes, a person with MTHFR gene defect should take a multivitamin especially formulated for MTHFR to improve the effectiveness of the antidepressant.

- BPD people cut themselves or become very abusive because the hormone released through cutting or expression of anger/frustration lowers the amplification of oxytocin level, and thus, they feel relief.

- Depressive person attempts suicide because they can't think rationally or clearly (very low glutamate) and to relieve their massive emotional pain (very low serotonin).

- As depression reflects a total inhibiting brain energy level, and we know that energy can be measured, it will truly be beneficial if there were an affordable & easy to use mobile application that can sense this energy through a sensor attached to a mobile phone. Hence, depression can be detected and prevented before it occurs.

Acknowledgement

This theory on men metabolic syndrome/infertility (MetS) and Depression (BPD/Borderline, Dysthymia, Bipolar, Major) was developed based on a few key concepts from:

a. Dr. Ameet Aggarwal, a naturopathic doctor whose work (http://drameet.com) helped the author to see that a health issue is primarily due to an imbalance body, mind and spirit. Thus, there are natural and holistic ways to heal from the imbalance. His book also helped the author to view the health imbalance from a bodily function perspective.

b. Dr. William Walsh, a mental health nutrition practitioner, whose research is freely available online (https://www.walshinstitute.org), helped the author to see that mental health problems can be quantifiable. His work also helped the author to view the health imbalance from a nutrition and gene perspective.

c. Thus, the initial theory was an amalgamation of the above 2 concepts, a natural and quantifiable approach to mental health. From here, another influential work is from Dr. Andrew L. Rostenberg, whose work is available on his website (http://www.beyondmthfr.com). His work helped the author to understand that mental health is not found at the extremes.

d. Dr. Brant Cortright, a professor of psychology, (http://www.brantcortright.com), whose work on neurogenesis gives hope and points to a solution for the mental health imbalance. It also helped the author to view mental health imbalance from an oxidation and neuron perspective.

e. Dr. Ben Lynch, a naturopathic doctor and MTHFR expert (http://mthfr.net), whose health supplements are a God send.

f. Professor Jayashri Kulkarni, a field leader in Borderline Personality Disorder and Polycystic Ovarian Syndrome (i.e. relates to metabolic/endocrine), whose work confirmed the link between these 2 seemingly disparate disorders.

g. Wikipedia contributors, honest testimonials from people, health researches, medical vloggers/bloggers and health vloggers/bloggers, who took the time to share and upload their work on the World Wide Web.

h. The author's family, whose battle with mental health propelled the author to find the root cause and solutions to their mental health challenge and in doing so, helped the author to discover the root cause and solutions to the author's own metabolic syndrome challenge.

i. Finally, above all, God, where we are all "***Fearfully and wonderfully made***". This gives hope that there is an intricate order and intelligence in our bodies to heal, as long as we find the root cause to our health imbalance. Therefore, our symptoms will no longer be fearful but instead, will be wonderful as God had intended.

Appendix 1: Links (*which are correct as of publishing date in Oct 2019*)

Link No	URL address
1	https://www.ncbi.nlm.nih.gov/pmc/articles/PMC6479081/
2	https://wjmh.org/Synapse/Data/PDFData/2074WJMH/wjmh-36-e37.pdf
3	https://www.ncbi.nlm.nih.gov/pmc/articles/PMC5003061/
4	https://www.researchgate.net/publication/38020165_Association_of_the_metabolic_syndrome_with_depression_and_anxiety_in_Japanese_men_A_1-year_cohort_study
5	https://www.ncbi.nlm.nih.gov/pmc/articles/PMC4309892/
6	https://pdfs.semanticscholar.org/44bd/c357b061976c0a059845d21fd10a06f9c5f7.pdf
7	https://www.meridianvalleylab.com/the-anticancer-testosterone-metabolite-3%CE%B2-adiol/
8	https://www.frontiersin.org/articles/10.3389/fendo.2015.00160/full
9	https://scanberlin.com/2016/05/26/oxytocin-the-story-of-a-misunderstood-hormone/
10	https://www.ncbi.nlm.nih.gov/pubmed/26231445
11	https://www.ncbi.nlm.nih.gov/pmc/articles/PMC3389841/#!po=0.666667
12	https://www.karger.com/article/fulltext/338397
13	http://www.jneurosci.org/content/26/5/1448
14	https://www.hindawi.com/journals/ije/2015/294278/
15	https://en.m.wikipedia.org/wiki/Aromatase
16	http://tau.amegroups.com/article/view/3516/4362
17	https://www.healthline.com/health/beauty-skin-care/pimple-acne-face-map#takeaway
18	https://www.ncbi.nlm.nih.gov/m/pubmed/29107881/
19	https://www.ncbi.nlm.nih.gov/pmc/articles/PMC3820276/
20	https://science.howstuffworks.com/life/inside-the-mind/emotions/bored-to-death1.htm
21	https://www.livestrong.com/article/528128-glutamine-gaba/
22	https://www.ncbi.nlm.nih.gov/pmc/articles/PMC5793728/
23	https://www.psychiatry.org/patients-families/dissociative-disorders/what-are-dissociative-disorders
24	http://www.borderlinecentral.com/articles/rootofbpd.php
25	http://www.borderlinecentral.com/articles/primaryrelationship.php
26	http://www.borderlinecentral.com/articles/bpdintimacyissue.php
27	http://www.borderlinecentral.com/articles/bpdrelationship.php
28	https://ipfs.io/ipfs/QmXoypizjW3WknFiJnKLwHCnL72vedxjQkDDP1mXWo6uco/wiki/Borderline_personality_disorder.html
29	http://www.borderlinecentral.com
30	https://www.psychologytoday.com/blog/matter-personality/201410/treatment-resistant-depression-and-borderline-personality
31	https://www.ncbi.nlm.nih.gov/pmc/articles/PMC4310835/
32	https://www.maurerfoundation.org/what-are-free-radicals/
33	https://www.ncbi.nlm.nih.gov/m/pubmed/19149749/
34	https://www.popsci.com/chronic-stress-causes-inflammation-in-brain
35	https://www.maurerfoundation.org/what-are-free-radicals/
36	https://www.ncbi.nlm.nih.gov/pmc/articles/PMC4307252/
37	http://www.buffalo.edu/news/releases/2000/08/4839.html
38	https://www.naturalendocrinesolutions.com/articles/methylation-mthfr-thyroid-health/
39	https://www.google.com/amp/s/amp.mindbodygreen.com/articles/methylation-why-it-matters-for-your-immunity-inflammation-more--18245
40	https://www.healthline.com/health/cortisol-urine#uses
41	http://www.buffalo.edu/news/releases/2000/08/4839.html
42	www.google.com/amp/s/amp.mindbodygreen.com/articles/gaba-what-is-it
43	https://neurohacker.com/what-is-glutamate
44	https://www.naturalgroarticle/glutamine-most-cers.com/versatile-amino-acid
45	https://media.cellsignal.com/www/pdfs/content-fragments/gu-nt2-amino-acid-poster.pdf

Link No	URL Address
46	https://onlinelibrary.wiley.com/doi/10.1177/0884533617691250
47	www.aminoacidsguide.com
48	https://www.teachengineering.org/lessons/view/cub_human_lesson07
49	http://www.cryst.bbk.ac.uk/pps97/assignments/projects/adomas/Free_Radical_Damages_In_Proteins.html
50	https://www.endocrineweb.com/conditions/type-2-diabetes/insulin-resistance-causes-symptoms
51	https://www.ncbi.nlm.nih.gov/m/pubmed/10342671/
52	https://care.diabetesjournals.org/content/34/7/1669
53	https://www.ncbi.nlm.nih.gov/pmc/articles/PMC2835908/
54	https://www.ncbi.nlm.nih.gov/pmc/articles/PMC3012032/
55	https://www.ncbi.nlm.nih.gov/m/pubmed/16778793/
56	https://www.ncbi.nlm.nih.gov/pmc/articles/PMC2835908/
57	https://www.ncbi.nlm.nih.gov/pmc/articles/PMC3051853/#!po=26.6917
58	https://www.physiology.org/doi/full/10.1152/ajpendo.00444.2007
59	https://www.ncbi.nlm.nih.gov/pubmed/8013750?dopt=Abstract
60	https://www.sciencedaily.com/releases/2010/06/100621091205.htm
61	https://www.ncbi.nlm.nih.gov/pmc/articles/PMC4565209/
62	https://www.medicaljournals.se/acta/download/10.2340/00015555-1677/
63	https://academic.oup.com/ajcn/article/86/1/107/4633089
64	https://www.ncbi.nlm.nih.gov/pubmed/12450882
65	https://www.labce.com/spg1094049_phase_i_reactions_hydrolysis_reduction_and_oxidati.aspx
66	https://www.ncbi.nlm.nih.gov/books/NBK22339/
67	https://en.m.wikipedia.org/wiki/Aromatase
68	http://tau.amegroups.com/article/view/3516/4362
69	https://www.webmd.com/men/features/infertility
70	https://www.ncbi.nlm.nih.gov/pubmed/24673246
71	https://www.sciencedirect.com/science/article/pii/S092544390900218X
72	https://www.ncbi.nlm.nih.gov/pmc/articlcs/PMC3074428/
73	https://academic.oup.com/jn/article/147/3/281/4584732
74	https://www.ncbi.nlm.nih.gov/m/pubmed/12416261/
75	https://www.ncbi.nlm.nih.gov/pmc/articles/PMC3449194/
76	https://www.ncbi.nlm.nih.gov/pmc/articles/PMC3354945/
77	https://www.ncbi.nlm.nih.gov/pmc/articles/PMC4708304/#!po=0.568182
78	https://www.webmd.com/men/features/infertility
79	https://www.ncbi.nlm.nih.gov/m/pubmed/3200122/
80	https://academic.oup.com/edrv/article/27/1/2/2355160
81	https://www.webmd.com/cholesterol-management/cholesterol-and-artery-plaque-buildup
82	https://www.kidney.org/atoz/content/Stress_and_your_Kidneys
83	https://www.aminoacid-studies.com/areas-of-use/cholesterol.html
84	https://news.illinois.edu/view/6367/204646
85	https://www.intechopen.com/books/soybean-bio-active-compounds/soybean-nutrition-and-health
86	http://www.buffalo.edu/news/releases/2000/08/4839.html
87	https://www.hindawi.com/journals/ije/2015/294278/
88	https://m.caltech.edu/about/news/microbes-help-produce-serotonin-gut-46495
89	https://bodyecology.com/articles/why_proper_bile_flow_essential_for_getting_rid_of_toxins-php/
90	https://www.integrativefamilypractice.com/blog/liver-detoxification
91	https://www.ncbi.nlm.nih.gov/books/NBK279393/#!po=34.6154
92	https://www.ncbi.nlm.nih.gov/books/NBK22339/
93	https://health.howstuffworks.com/diseases-conditions/cardiovascular/cholesterol/difference-between-ldl-and-hdl-cholesterol.htm

Radical theory on MetS & Depression

Link No	URL Address
94	https://www.livestrong.com/article/252226-triglycerides-and-digestion/
95	https://www.medicalnewstoday.com/articles/322017.php
96	http://www.vivo.colostate.edu/hbooks/pathphys/digestion/liver/bile.html
97	https://www.health.harvard.edu/heart-health/how-its-made-cholesterol-production-in-your-body
98	https://www.womensinternational.com/portfolio-items/liver/
99	https://www.hindawi.com/journals/ije/2015/294278/
100	https://www.samanthagilbert.com/glutamine-is-this-powerful-nutrient-safe-for-you/
101	https://dutchtest.com
102	https://www.spectracell.com
103	https://www.nutripath.com.au
104	https://www.sciencedirect.com/science/article/pii/S2213158216302467
105	https://www.ncbi.nlm.nih.gov/pmc/articles/PMC2837268/#!po=25.3769
106	https://dmm.biologists.org/content/5/6/746
107	https://www.ncbi.nlm.nih.gov/pmc/articles/PMC3074630/#!po=5.44872
108	https://www.ncbi.nlm.nih.gov/m/pubmed/23306210/
109	https://www.frontiersin.org/articles/10.3389/fnins.2014.00130/full
110	https://www.sciencedaily.com/releases/2008/08/080831114717.htm
111	https://www.lifeextension.com/Magazine/2017/8/Brant-Cortright-Phd-The-Neurogenesis-Diet-and-Lifestyle/Page-01
112	https://www.tandfonline.com/doi/pdf/10.1179/135100003225003393
113	https://en.m.wikipedia.org/wiki/Glutamate_receptor
114	https://www.ncbi.nlm.nih.gov/m/pubmed/19207807/
115	https://en.m.wikipedia.org/wiki/Dopamine_receptor
116	https://www.ncbi.nlm.nih.gov/m/pubmed/17088501/
117	https://www.ncbi.nlm.nih.gov/pmc/articles/PMC4942262/
118	https://www.sciencedirect.com/topics/social-sciences/serotonin
119	https://nutritiongenome.com/what-is-comt/
120	http://www.beyondmthfr.com/treating-comt-and-mao-how-comt-influences-the-brain/).
121	https://www.ncbi.nlm.nih.gov/pubmed/23668908
122	https://www.frontiersin.org/articles/10.3389/fpsyt.2016.00156/full
123	https://www.ncbi.nlm.nih.gov/pmc/articles/PMC5831952/
124	https://en.m.wikipedia.org/wiki/Apathy
125	https://www.sciencedaily.com/releases/2013/07/130722123206.htm
126	http://sitn.hms.harvard.edu/flash/2017/love-actually-science-behind-lust-attraction-companionship/
127	https://www.medicalnewstoday.com/articles/271544.php
128	https://www.ncbi.nlm.nih.gov/pubmed/18950248
129	https://www.mja.com.au/system/files/issues/001_04_011012/bea10474_fm.pdf
130	https://www.ncbi.nlm.nih.gov/pubmed/18950248
131	https://www.ncbi.nlm.nih.gov/pubmed/20676614
132	https://drjockers.com/gaba/
133	http://www.rlcure.com/glutamate2.html
134	https://universityhealthnews.com/daily/depression/borderline-personality-disorder-treatment-research-promising-for-natural-omega-3/
135	https://www.sciencedirect.com/science/article/pii/S092544390900218X
136	https://www.ncbi.nlm.nih.gov/pmc/articles/PMC2556928/pdf/ehp0108-000867.pdf
137	https://ipfs.io/ipfs/QmXoypizjW3WknFiJnKLwHCnL72vedxjQkDDP1mXWo6uco/wiki/Borderline_personality_disorder.html
138	https://www.verywellmind.com/effect-of-hormones-on-social-anxiety-4129255
139	https://www.medicalnewstoday.com/articles/amp/323712
140	https://jamanetwork.com/journals/jamapsychiatry/article-abstract/2712976
141	https://www.avogel.co.uk/herbal-remedies/milk-thistle/

Link No	URL Address
142	https://universityhealthnews.com/daily/depression/best-probiotics-for-mood-enhancing-the-gut-brain-connection-with-psychobiotics/
143	https://gohealthy.co.nz/products/general-health/probiotic-75-billion/
144	https://www.seekinghealth.com/collections/multivitamins

www.ingramcontent.com/pod-product-compliance
Lightning Source LLC
Chambersburg PA
CBHW051156220526
45473CB00003B/789